Inside Laboratory Medicine

T0197953

Inside Laboratory Medicine

A Memoir of Healthcare Behind the Scenes

Nyla Jo Hubbard

McFarland & Company, Inc., Publishers

Jefferson, North Carolina

ISBN (print) 978-1-4766-9565-5
ISBN (ebook) 978-1-4766-5328-0

LIBRARY OF CONGRESS AND BRITISH LIBRARY
CATALOGUING DATA ARE AVAILABLE

Library of Congress Control Number 2024017217

Front cover: (top inset) the author in a hospital lab, circa 2000;
(bottom) photograph of a petri dish by Anna Ivanova (Shutterstock)

Printed in the United States of America

*McFarland & Company, Inc., Publishers
Box 611, Jefferson, North Carolina 28640
www.mcfarlandpub.com*

To the many technicians, technologists and aides who work every day in clinical laboratories, often located in a windowless basement and visited only by co-workers and the occasional doctor or nurse. There are about 260,000 CLIA certified laboratories in the U.S. and 14 billion laboratory tests are ordered annually. The laboratory provides 70 percent of the data the doctor uses to diagnose and treat patients (CDC D. o., 2018), but laboratory techs are almost never seen. We remain sequestered and unknown to patients. This is your story and the story of all techs like you.

Table of Contents

Table of Contents

Preface

I decided to write this book during the Covid pandemic. I kept hearing about the doctors, nurses and EMTs who were working with Covid patients. They were being called heroes and rightly so, but it was obvious that the general public was not aware of who was actually running all of those Covid tests. Laboratorians were never mentioned. It brought home to me the fact that the public and even the patients using lab services do not know who we are and what we do in the clinical lab. I spoke to other techs and it surfaced that we would all like to have our story told. Though unseen, we are an integral part of the healthcare team.

I have used pseudonyms for techs mentioned in this book unless I was able to get signed releases allowing me to use their full names. The book covers forty years of laboratory experience in different kinds of labs: clinics, hospitals, reference labs and even my mission as a lab tech with Doctors Without Borders in Ethiopia. I have covered the methods we used to employ as well as the updated ways of testing. Moreover, I have included patient stories, the human side of laboratory medicine. Several techs were kind enough to participate in interviews and to tell me what being a tech has meant to them. A recurring comment was that, though they knew they were necessary to the care of the patient, they did not feel that their work was acknowledged by anyone beyond their own peers. In this book, I bring them out of the shadows and allow them to tell their story.

Prologue

The Coulter counter clicked like a Geiger counter finding uranium. My coworker and I glanced at each other across the small clinic lab. Accustomed as we were to the more sedate clicking of a normal white cell count, it was startling. I immediately thought that maybe it was a contaminant in the sample. At that time, we diluted our samples by hand and washed the plastic cuvettes for reuse. Our delivery man, in this case, the patient, was sitting right there in the drawing chair, watching the proceedings. He came in that day with his delivery and an order he had procured from one of our inhouse doctors for a CBC, that is, Complete Blood Count. He told us he had been feeling somewhat tired.

I carefully diluted another aliquot (measured amount) of blood with the proper amount of sterile diluent. Once again, the clicking was manic. I went to the slide, a film of blood prepared by deftly using another glass slide to form a thin film of blood only one cell thick at the edges. It had been stained with the requisite Wright stain. One glance was all I needed. Chuck, our jovial delivery man, had leukemia. His WBC (white blood cell count) was nearly 100,000 when normal for him would have been no more than 11,000 (Merck, 2022). There were also immature white cells on his slide, lots of them.

One of the first things we learn when training as techs is to hide any shocking results from the patient. That news should be given by a doctor in a contained situation. I simply told him I would give the doctor the results. I later asked the doctor about Chuck's response after being seen. Our doctor said he had arranged for a hematologist closer to Chuck's home to see him for follow-up. I never learned the outcome. It is one of the frustrations of being sequestered in the lab. We often do not learn what happens next. Given the treatment options in 1968, I'm afraid it wasn't good. But at least he was diagnosed and offered a chance thanks to laboratory training and experience.

ONE

Beginning:
The Clinical Lab in 1968

I worked in the clinical lab for more than forty years but, too often, when I told people that I was a lab tech, they said, "Oh, you draw blood."

In general, techs don't draw blood anymore. In most places, phlebotomists, including those called Medical Laboratory Assistants, have taken over that duty. Even when we went out on the floors to draw, that was only a prerequisite to the work waiting for us back in the lab. There are thousands of lab tests, dozens of different laboratory computer systems, hundreds of different instruments and a small army of highly trained technicians, technologists and supervisors who have to learn to master all of the above. They are almost all truly dedicated individuals who work all shifts, holidays and weekends so that your doctor gets your results in a timely manner. Many credit hours of science are required before they even start learning the technical side of lab work as it is important to understand what you are doing in order to do it right.

I have often wondered who patients think is running those tests. If they are curious, they probably think the doctors and interns are in there doing the tests themselves. That is not the case. I think patients would be truly amazed if they stepped behind those laboratory doors and saw the lab coated worker bees in front of their multi-million-dollar instruments, peering down their microscopes, reading their culture plates, slicing and staining tumor samples or crossmatching blood as fast as it is possible to go. In these pages, I will introduce you.

I suppose it was fore destined that I would ultimately work in the lab. I was the only girl in my high school biology class who actually liked dissection. I was fascinated with the internal anatomy of the chickens we killed and dressed on the farm in Indiana where I grew up and I cut open a dead garter snake just to see what was inside. My great-aunt was head nurse at Marion General Hospital and I was very impressed by her navy blue cloak with its red lining, her starched cap and spiffy uniform. I might have gone into nursing if I hadn't developed Henoch-Schonlein purpura at the age of five. This condition affects mostly young children. I remember that my hands swelled up and I had an extensive rash. I'm told that I had bleeding into the stomach and kidneys. We never learned the cause and the condition resolved itself. In the hospital in Indianapolis, I was given plasma in one of those old-fashioned glass bottles and was required to visit the laboratory for bleeding time tests thereafter. In 1950, the method was to prick an earlobe rather than the fingertip and I listened to the tech explain to my mother that they would be looking at the number of my platelets. I visualized tiny dinner plates circulating though my body. Who wouldn't be intrigued by lab work after that experience?

Money was always an issue in my childhood home. No one had ever been to college. My parents did have respect for education but, as was so often the case in the 1950s and 1960s, it was not assumed that girls would go into the sciences. My parents were known to say to me, "Oh, you'll just get married and have kids." I don't know why they made this assumption since my mother worked outside the home for most of her life but that was the mindset at the time. I did marry and had a two-year-old son when the opportunity presented itself to begin work in the lab. I met a woman who worked in the kitchen of our local hospital. I mentioned that my son was old enough now for daycare and I really wanted (and needed) to go to work but I wanted to work in medicine. She said the lab director was looking for techs and he was willing to train someone inhouse who would also take on other tasks. It was a paid position—but not much.

I applied and was given the position. We were expected to wear white uniforms at the time and white shoes. We did not yet have white lab coats. I began with running EKGs since, at that time, they were under the auspices of the laboratory. It wasn't difficult, though the small 50-bed hospital was overloaded and I often had to run EKGs on patients who lay in beds in the hall with just a curtain drawn around the both of us. I was careful with the curtain because a uniform dress was not the best choice of attire when bending over beds in the hall. I often felt as exposed as the patients.

The machines back then were clunky and had none of the stick-on leads that are used now. Instead, we had weighted belts that were supposed to hold the leads in place. It took some maneuvering to arrange the belt so that it held the leads tightly on a sloping body. Of course, I got better at positioning and I enjoyed getting to know the patients. I remember some to this day fifty-five years later! There was the beekeeper who had his hive fall off the bed of his pickup truck when he was trying to load it. He had hundreds of stings but he said he didn't blame the bees. He still loved them.

There was the multiple myeloma patient who had open bed sores which gave off a terrible smell. I felt so sorry for this lady who had indescribable bone pain from the illness and then had to suffer open sores and watch people hold their breath when they came into the room. It gave me the opportunity to see the living patient with this condition before I later learned the pathology.

We had one patient with tertiary (third stage) syphilis, a condition I have never seen since. Syphilis is caused by a spiral shaped bacteria called *Treponema pallidum.* This man had contracted the disease many years before but had never been adequately treated. By this time, it had caused dementia and blindness, a good reminder that the old diseases are still around.

I think the gravity of a job in medicine was first impressed upon me when I was called to the ER to run an EKG on my first Code Blue. A Code Blue is a genuine emergency. The patient's heart is not functioning and no oxygen is reaching the brain. In this case, the patient was only 45 years old and had already visited his family doctor when he had trouble breathing and pain going down his left arm. The doctor sent him to us and, about the time I rolled my cart into the room, he went into full arrest. I hooked up the machine and placed the electrodes in the proper positions but the graph on the tape coming out of the machine was like none I had seen before. The nurse on duty quickly placed a tongue depressor between the patient's teeth as he appeared to go into seizure. The ER doctor ordered defibrillation and they shocked this poor man more than once without success. Unbelievable to me, this youngish man, who had been talking and breathing just moments before, was pronounced dead.

The staff cleaned up and suggested we go to break. I was shocked. I had never seen someone die. "Break," I thought! How can we possibly drink coffee and eat breakfast after this experience? I knew his wife was sitting in the waiting room, completely unaware. It was unthinkable. The nurse, who became a friend, saw my distress. "We have to eat," she told me, "There will be other patients, other emergencies, and we have to be ready for them."

Some techs today do not learn to draw blood, but I trained before the advent of phlebotomists and we drew a lot of it. I started on patients just out of surgery when they were safely "out of it" and couldn't complain. I think anyone is understandably squeamish when they first insert a needle into a real live arm. Of course, I was told which veins to use and it was demonstrated, but it is a skill which takes practice and I worked hard to be good at it. We also had to learn which tube to use as each color is for a different type of test. The purple topped tubes contain an anticoagulant called EDTA so the blood will not clot and is the right tube for hematology. Protimes, short for prothrombin, a test for clotting time, use a different anticoagulant and chemistries use blood that is clotted, spun down and the serum removed so red topped tubes have no anticoagulant.

My other duties, as a paid trainee, included tabulating charges and washing glassware. There was a great deal of that since it was before so many disposables came on the scene. In the afternoons, we hit the books. My supervisor was a lech. Clinical labs have been around for at least 200 years, beginning mainly in Germany, France and England (Buttner, 1992). Women were probably always used as assistants and indeed, when I began working, almost all the techs were women and virtually all the supervisors were men. Today, he could be charged in the "meToo" movement due to his penchant for putting his arms on either side of me when I was at the scope, pinning me against him. He wasn't above putting his arms around me through the curtains when I had them pulled around a patient bed, either. But I really wanted to work so I put up with him like everyone else did. Having to tolerate this injustice was only one issue in 1968. A woman couldn't get a mortgage or a credit card in her own name unless a husband or a father cosigned. Yes, it's incredible but true, just fifty scant years ago. We all recognized the wrong but we had not yet come together to make our voices heard.

I'm not sure he hired me for the right reasons but he was a smart man and he chose the books I needed to buy with care. I had always done well in school, a trait I think I share with many techs, since the material is complex and requires real concentration. We began with hematology.

There is a hierarchy in the clinical lab. The first rung is technician, then technologist, then supervisor. At that time, I was earning the right to sit the exam for a technician. The state of Florida had recently instituted licensure requirements. The technician exam encompassed all the departments in the lab, though not at the advanced level of a technologist. Hematology means literally the "study of the blood." I learned the backup methods first. Labs must have such backups, as machines go down but lives still depend on results. Red cell and white cell pipettes had been used for many years. They were calibrated devices using a small amount of blood mixed in a small glass cylinder specific for the task. The blood was mixed with a diluent, plated on a special counting chamber and the cells were counted under the microscope. No other machinery was needed but it required great care in making the dilution and was a slow process.

When people are ill or dying, the results can't wait. Enter Coulter counters which made it possible to get results out sooner. They were fairly new in 1968 and were used only for white cell counts and red cell counts. The principle behind the machine is the use of a laser beam which is interrupted when a cell passes through the tiny aperture. When I began training, the red cell counts were done on a dilution of whole blood and white cell counts were done separately and required a lysing agent which eliminated the red cells so that only white cells passed through the aperture. The total white blood cell count is important but it doesn't tell the whole story. The white cells of the blood are varied. There are the neutrophils which seek out bacterial invaders and phagocytize (from the Latin "to eat") them, the lymphocytes which are also varied but are involved in the immune system, and the monocytes, which do the cleanup after the neutrophils have attacked the enemy. Eosinophils carry histamine, which is involved in allergic reactions and is the reason we take antihistamines to combat the symptoms. Eos are also increased in parasitic infections. Lastly, there are the basophils, which are few in number but are also involved in response to inflammation.

The normal for a WBC count is 4,500–11,000 per microliter (1,000,000th of a liter) of whole blood (Merck, 2022). It goes up in response to many infections, particularly bacterial infections. That is why it is a good indicator for whether to give antibiotics or not. However, a complete blood count also requires tabulating the types of white cells seen under the microscope because immature neutrophils, called stabs or bands, are increased in bacterial infection, sometimes even before the total WBC count goes up. I found this to be particularly true in children. Lymphocytes are often increased in viral infections and the

9

total WBC count can be decreased in this type of illness. We count 100 white blood cells under the scope, tabulating by using different keys on the "diff" counter (or today on the computer keyboard) for each type of cell. This is called a differential, "diff" for short. The first thing we learn is to recognize the normal cells. If you have a thorough grasp of what a normal cell looks like, you will instantly recognize an abnormal cell.

A normal red cell count is 4.2 million to 5.9 million cells per microliter of blood (Merck, 2022). The count can be reduced by anemia, bleeding, or a variety of abnormal conditions. It is increased in polycythemia. That is not good for the patient as the blood is thicker and harder for the heart to pump. When we do the differential, we are also looking at the red cells because there are many conditions in which the red cells are not normal. Mature human red cells have no nucleus, having lost it as they matured in the bone marrow. They are disc shaped and appear under the scope as having a central pallor where they are thin in the center. They can have inclusions. It is not so common now, but I used to see indication of lead ingestion in children in the red cells before lead paint was banned. Malaria parasites show up in red blood cells.

Platelets are remnants of the mother cells, megakaryocytes, which are formed in the bone marrow and fragment, giving us one important factor in the clotting of blood. It is important to make sure adequate platelets appear in the blood smear and the size is noted.

It was hard work in those early days. I had to learn many new things including the different types of glassware. We had graduated flasks which are tall and cylindrical with many gradations, Erlenmeyer flasks, which are wide at the bottom and narrow at the top, and volumetric flasks which hold only a specified volume. With all the flasks, I had to learn about the meniscus which is the crescent shape formed by a liquid at the surface. We read the bottom of the meniscus for accuracy. There were various glass pipettes, tubes which are, like flasks, either graduated or volumetric. If a pipette got stopped up, we had stylets to clean them. I had to wash all of these using an apparatus we attached to the faucet at the sink and I had to get all my paid work done in order to have time for classroom instruction. But it was a joy because everything was new and I was becoming part of a team. This is a very important part of lab work because outsiders do not normally see us and we are excluded from the well-recognized coterie of doctors, nurses, therapists that do hands-on care. We rely on each other in the lab and I will be forever grateful to those techs who taught me.

I also had all the doubts and feelings of inadequacy about leaving my two-year-old son in daycare. He had far too many bumps and bruises at the first place I tried so I moved him to a "nursery school" so close to the hospital that I could see his bright blond head moving around in the play yard when I was in the break room and he was outside. He loved playing with the other kids and I told myself that I was preparing to provide for him better later on. I wasn't doing much in the way of providing at the time as the childcare, a big $20 per week, took about half of my paycheck.

Every lab in Florida must be headed by a pathologist, a "doctor of disease." They are physicians first who then go on to specialize in pathology. It is a pathologist who decides if your specimen shows signs of cancer or whether the cells in your sample could be leukemia. They normally see patients only when performing a bone marrow biopsy or an autopsy but they are always there behind the scenes, and they are our go to resource in the lab.

Our pathologist when I began training was a Dr. Smith. He was from Indiana as was I, and he often would break into singing "On the Banks of the Wabash" when he saw me. Dr. Smith made a point of including us in unusual diagnoses and we gathered around for any teaching moment. I well remember the lesson involving a smoker's lung. He showed us the fresh, pink, spongy tissue of a healthy lung contrasted with the black, solid-looking lung of a recently deceased smoker. I didn't smoke and I knew I wouldn't start after that lesson.

Of course, in the past, I had only known doctors in a patient capacity. In the hospital, I was often delegated to carry lab results to physicians since this was in the days before computers made everything instantly accessible. One day, I delivered a lab slip to a Dr. O. He had a Germanic name which was hard to pronounce so we called him by the initial. I don't know if he was from Germany or only of German descent, but he was a tall, formidable doctor with a stern expression and always wore a long white, well-starched coat. I had been washing glassware for some time and had developed an allergy to the soap. My hands looked like hamburger and itched unmercifully but I was so determined to finish my training, I had not complained. When I handed Dr. O the slip, he grabbed my hand and said, "What's this?"

I told him about the allergy and he said, "Come with me." Off we went to Central Supply where he insisted that the clerk give me a tube of Kenalog cream. Little did I know that I had just been introduced to the first cortisone cream on the market. The cream truly worked miracles and it reconfirmed my faith that the majority of doctors really care about relieving suffering, including mine.

After I had mastered basic hematology, we moved on to chemistry. I began to see the correlation between the abnormal EKGs I was running and the elevated CK (creatine kinase) results on the same patients. This enzyme is released from damaged heart muscle and was the best indicator we had at the time for substantiating a heart attack. We ran other enzymes such as amylase to diagnose pancreatitis. We had to master using a bulb to draw the serum (the fluid portion of the blood left after clotting) into the pipette because there is amylase in saliva. For other tests, we mouth pipetted, meaning we drew the fluid up in the pipette by sucking with our mouths. One reagent was picric acid for running creatinine. It was a mustard yellow fluid which was poisonous but we all blithely pipetted it by mouth and I don't think I ever realized how dangerous the stuff was until Midge, a fellow tech, told me of her experience with it.

This was during the 1970s before an inspection. The techs were cleaning out the cabinets. This had not been done for years. They found a sizable bottle of picric acid which had begun to dry out. The supervisor called for someone to remove it and the next thing they knew, they had orders to evacuate the lab while hazmat people in their white suits came in to carry out the picric acid. It turned out that picric acid in dry form will explode. It was a good thing they had decided to clean house or it might have continued to dry out until it blew off the cabinet doors and caused injury. Today, reagents are more safely packaged and mouth pipetting is forbidden for obvious reasons since it exposed us to disease and various chemicals.

I had to learn to think in metrics and Celsius temperature as only those units are used in the laboratory. After I got used to it, I realized how much easier it is to convert from volume to mass, etc., using metric units rather than English units. We also used the 24-hour clock. Five o'clock in the afternoon became 1700 hours. I enjoyed the specificity of it all.

One of the most challenging techniques to learn was the drawing and using of logarithmic curves. Volumetric tests such as sugars, BUNs (blood urea nitrogen) or creatinine (for kidney function) required dilution by hand with a reagent specific to the test and the use of a colorimeter, a machine that read the depth of color formed in the solution.

More sugar, etc., equaled more color. A curve was formulated by using standards. These were known amounts of the substance in question, bought from a company. We ran graduated dilutions of the standard and got our colorimeter readings. We then used big log paper to make a graph, with colorimeter reading on one axis and the amount of the analyte contained in the dilution on the other axis. Where the two intersected made a point. A line was drawn connecting these points, forming a curve. We then used the colorimeter readings from patient samples to find the amount of glucose, etc., from this curve. Of course, the dilutions had to be exact and there were several of them for each analyte (type of test). A new curve had to be run every time we got a new batch of reagent since every batch could be slightly different and would affect the results. There was always a certain amount of tension involved when setting up a new curve because if the points did not "line up" we had to start over. If the level of glucose or other analyte in a sample was higher than the highest standard, the sample had to be diluted to be able to read it off the curve.

Another source of worry for me was using the flame photometer. We used this instrument to measure electrolytes. Electrolytes such as sodium (Na), potassium (K), chloride (Cl) and CO_2 are absolutely crucial to the functioning of the human body. The exchange of ions across cell membranes is what makes your muscles work, including the heart muscle. Medications, diabetes, dehydration, or kidney disease can alter the levels of electrolytes and they are one of the most commonly ordered "stat" tests (stat means "immediately") in the lab. The flame setup required big cylinders of oxygen and I found the lighting of it to be scary but I had to learn.

The principle behind using a flame is that each of the elements gives off a distinct wavelength of light when vaporized. Sodium gives off a yellow light and potassium gives off purple. Colored filters made it possible to isolate one from the other and the amount of light emitted was converted to a numerical result. Chloride could be titrated and CO_2 was read with a complicated apparatus called a Van Slyke manometer. I look back on those fussy methods and think how much easier it was to get results later on with new technology. However, the volume of tests became so much higher later, with the increased population, lab work didn't get easier.

In addition to the colorimeter, we had a spectrophotometer. This instrument read in the UV range and was used to measure enzyme activity. We began by adding patient serum to a substrate specific to that enzyme, such as amylase or CK. As the enzyme present in the sample began to "eat" the substrate, more UV light could pass through. By taking readings sequentially, we could tell how much light passed through before and after the reaction and calculate how much of the enzyme was present in the sample.

I'm not sure that I would have stuck it out had the tension of constantly learning been unrelieved but there were other moments. A senior tech who was given the task of showing me how to do my first parasite exam did not like parasitology nor the awful smell that went with it since we did not have hoods with HEPA filters available in labs today.

Pauline came to the bench with 4×4 gauze squares shoved up her nose in a walrus imitation while she showed me how to do the zinc flotation method of trying to find parasite eggs in a stool sample. I admit to being a bit put off. Somehow, I had only associated testing with blood or urine, not stool? I soon realized that it went with the territory and I had been raised on the farm so manure wasn't new.

Another memorable moment was when another tech accidentally set her hair on fire while using a flame to sterilize her loop when setting up cultures. She raced out of the back room with hair aflame but, before any of us could move, a person from accounting entered the main lab door, assessed the situation immediately, and used his hands to put out the fire. He was not burnt and she had only some singed tresses.

We moved on from chemistry to blood bank, a vastly different discipline. I had to learn to group and type blood. Your group is O, A, B or AB. Your type is Rh positive or negative. After a patient's blood is grouped and typed, it is crossmatched with a donor unit if a crossmatch is ordered. Normally, this is a pretty simple, though very careful, process but many people develop antibodies or are born with them and that particular donor blood may react and cannot be given safely to that particular patient. A primary example of a developed antibody is seen in Rh negative women who bear Rh positive infants. There is some "leak" of baby cells into the mother's bloodstream during pregnancy and an antibody to the Rh factor in her baby's blood develops in her own. The first Rh positive baby is usually OK but the body remembers and it will attack any future Rh positive infants while in utero and they can suffer from the condition called erythroblastosis fetalis. The condition can result in miscarriage. Babies born with this condition can be jaundiced, are likely to be anemic and can even die.

It was once necessary to transfuse the entire blood supply of an affected baby immediately after or even before birth to counteract this reaction. Thankfully, medical science came up with what could be called a "vaccine" named RhoGAM. It is given to any Rh negative mother if the father is Rh positive. It fools the body into thinking that it already has made an antibody so it won't make any more and vaccinated Rh negative women have had subsequent Rh positive infants without incident ever since. I used to wonder why, in my grandmother's family, every sister had only one child, quite unusual in the early 1900s. I later learned that they were all Rh negative and no doubt spontaneously aborted any subsequent pregnancies, probably before they knew they were pregnant.

The same reaction happens if an Rh negative patient of either sex is given Rh positive blood, perhaps in an emergency. One unit may not cause side effects but any further units of Rh positive blood will precipitate a serious reaction, quite possibly fatal. Lab work is not for the slapdash. Wrong results can damage or kill.

We drew donors in this lab and I had to learn to take blood pressures and temperatures as well as running hemoglobins on these donors as we made sure, as much as possible, that the donor was healthy. There were two big reclining chairs that patients sat in while we drew 500 ml. (roughly a pint) of blood. The needle was an 18 gauge, larger than the 21 gauge we usually used to draw blood samples, and I was squeamish the first few times I had to use this large needle for drawing donors but the needles were very sharp and they all lived through it. Donors were always given orange juice or a soft drink after the blood had been drawn to replace blood volume and to give them some sugar for energy. The blood they donated would be replaced quickly, the plasma within 24 hours and the red cells within weeks. The Red Cross recommends that people can give blood about every eight weeks if they are in good health (Cross, 2023).

We did not pay donors. That practice could be dangerous as people who had a communicable disease or were drug addicts had been known to sell their blood and whatever was in that blood could be passed on to the recipient. There was no big clearinghouse for blood as there is now and we mostly used what we drew inhouse. Today, there is much better testing of blood products and transfusion has become safer.

The other department of the lab was histology. Histo is a specialized branch and usually techs working in that department do not work anywhere else. It is an important part of the lab, however, because tissue samples and Pap smears are prepared and stained in Histo for the pathologists to read. It is here that the paths decide if the patient has cancer or another disease after the specimen has been properly sliced or stained for macroscopic and microscopic examination. I never worked in Histo but Histo techs fill a critical need in patient care.

Much has changed in forty years but the underlying principles remain the same and techs today face some of the same challenges. One thing that has not improved is access to affordable childcare. It's even more of a problem today than in 1968. The U.S. Department of Health and Human Services declares that childcare should take no more than 10 percent of a family's household budget. We wish! If I had been paying childcare on two children at the time I retired, given my rate of pay at that time, childcare would have been costing me almost a third of my wages, yet we seem to make no headway on instituting universal childcare. Mothers in the lab today still have to worry about where they are leaving their kids in order to take care of other people (Quicken, 2015).

Interview with a New Tech (2023)

Name, shift and duties, how long have you worked in the lab?

My name is Sam (short for Samantha) Lette. I trained at Erwin Technical School as an MLT (medical laboratory technician), and am now doing my internship during the day at a mid-size hospital lab. At Erwin, we got mostly theory. I did learn to draw blood and we learned the safety protocols that OSHA mandates. I also got the basics in hematology, chemistry and micro but I am learning a lot more now from the other techs. I really like it.

What is the biggest challenge for you in your job?

I will be on night shift when I finish my internship. I want to be able to troubleshoot the instruments and to organize my work for maximum productivity because I may be working alone and I haven't worked alone yet. I have to drive some distance to get to this job but it's worth it because it is a good learning environment. I think that is a must for a new tech.

Is your job different since Covid? How did it affect you during the epidemic?

I did not experience Covid but I've heard about it. I heard about the N95 masks and I know it may not be the last epidemic.

Do you feel stressed in your job? If so, do you have some on-the-job support?

I haven't experienced stress yet. I know that there will be people I can call if I feel overwhelmed.

How does your work affect home life? Do you find it difficult to balance work and home? How do you handle childcare, if applicable?

I'm not married and don't have kids yet so I don't have those worries. I think I will be OK on night shift because I've always been a night owl. I don't go to bed early so I think I'll be able to adjust to that shift.

Do you feel that you are recognized as part of the healthcare team?

Yes. But I find that it is hard to explain to friends exactly what I do. I find that I am rambling on and they don't understand. People are

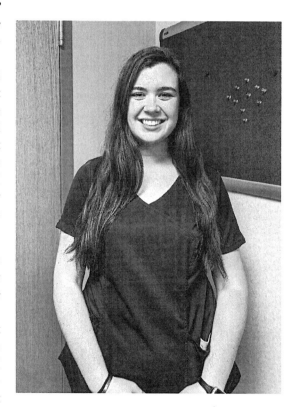

Samantha Lette, MLT

really unaware that there is a whole field of medicine, laboratory medicine, that they never see.

Do you feel satisfaction in your work? Are you glad you went into the field?

Yes. I originally started nursing but I was too empathetic for that. I then looked into forensic science but I found out that most of that work was onsite. I don't like working outside so I knew that wasn't for me. This is still in the medical field but a better fit.

Would you recommend young people go into this field? Why or why not? What would you tell them about the field?

Yes. I had the idea that all lab people would be quiet and reclusive but that isn't true. Different personalities come together in the lab but I do think it's important to be detail-oriented and a good multi-tasker because you will be doing more than one thing at a time.

Two

Meet the Patients: Clinic Work

I left that hospital when I became pregnant with my second child. My husband was very concerned that I would become "contaminated" with some germ. He was not a medical person and had never wanted me to work anyway. I was out of the lab for about four years. During that time, I took the test and passed it to receive my technician's license. I also started college courses as I wanted to move up the hierarchy ladder to medical technologist.

My next job was in a small medical clinic one county north. It did not pay as well as a hospital lab but tech pay almost anywhere was abysmal at that time. I made $1.40/hr. at the clinic, but I did not have to work holidays and weekends as I would have in a hospital. That was important as childcare was not available at those times. There were only two techs in our small lab and we took turns. One day I would do the blood draws and she would begin right away on the bench work. The next day we would switch. There were very busy days where I might draw up to forty patients and I learned the origin of the expression "vampire back." One unfortunate side effect of being a vampire came to light when I ran into a little girl in the grocery store whom I had drawn in the lab. She immediately crawled under the cart and scrunched herself up to avoid me. It made me feel like the enemy. The child recognized me, even without the short white lab coats we wore in the clinic.

I found out quickly, when I was doing the drawing, why we kept an ampoule of smelling salts next to the drawing chair. It was all too common for patients, often young men, to pass out during or after a blood draw. A young girl might tell me that she felt faint so I could get her head down and prevent a full faint. But young men did not like to admit that they were feeling ill and I had one who got up from the chair after the draw, only to have his knees buckle under him and down he went, out cold, taking up most of our floor space. I soon learned to advise people that, if it made them uncomfortable, to look away during the draw.

The assays were pretty simple but the atmosphere was different. We had three doctors and two PAs (physician assistants). Each had a nurse and there were two secretaries and various front office people. I saw all these people every day so I wasn't sequestered from the patients and the other caregivers as we were in the hospital. I loved it. The same patients came back year after year and we got to know them. We had a pass-through window for urine. The patient would urinate in the cup, open the little door on his or her side and place the urine sample on the platform between his door and ours. Then we simply opened the door on our side and retrieved the sample.

I remember instructing an elderly gentleman who was very hard of hearing on the procedure of how to collect a clean catch urine. It is important to get a "clean catch" urine so that you are reporting what is actually in the bladder, not on outside skin. The technique is to have the patient wipe around the opening to the urethra with a disinfectant wipe, hold the labia open in the case of a female patient, let a little urine go in the toilet, then catch the urine midstream in the cup. I was patiently explaining this system to the patient. He kept cupping his ear to show me he wasn't hearing but I finally thought he had understood what I was saying. Apparently, he did not. When I opened the door on my side of the pass-through window, he had put his hearing aide in the cup.

Urinalysis is not given the importance it deserves. My fellow tech, Judy, was told by a doctor that the good lord made women with the holes too close together. He meant that it is so easy for a female to infect her bladder by wiping stool with all the bacteria therein onto the opening of her urethra. I began to advise any (especially elderly) lady who came in with recurrent infections to make sure she wiped from front to back, not the other way round. It was amazing how many had never been told that fact.

When I have had a UTI (urinary tract infection), I have been thoroughly miserable but not everyone has recognizable symptoms. If the infection isn't caught early, it can go into the kidneys or even into the bloodstream causing septicemia. Urine gives us clues about other diseases as well. Sugar will show up in the urine and is often the way diabetes is first diagnosed. Bilirubin is another substance that alerts the doctor. Red cells may be undergoing damage elsewhere in the body and bilirubin is the byproduct. The specific gravity (density) of urine tells us when the patient is dehydrated, as the urine gets too concentrated. Most commonly, we look for white cells, blood, bacteria or yeast indicating infection. Various crystals can be seen in urine. Many are innocuous but some have real significance and can diagnose conditions such as gout. Parasites such as trichomonas can be detected in urine.

I learned patience working in the clinic. One day I was very busy and decided to instruct the female patient about her urine collection through the pass-through window rather than going out into the hall and bringing her into the bathroom. I pushed both doors open into the bathroom and called her name but she didn't see my face through the window. She was looking all over for me, behind the toilet, behind the wastepaper basket, everywhere except the window. I can't imagine how she thought anything larger than a fairy could be in those places but it was a lesson for me. After that, I went out and got the patients and instructed them onsite.

Though the tests we did were basic, we discovered serious conditions, such as the one I described in our deliveryman with leukemia. There was also a young boy, only 17, who came in for a football physical. I thought he looked pale and my observation was borne out by a low hemoglobin. Hemoglobin is the oxygen-carrying molecule contained in red cells. It has an iron component. We did hemoglobins by pipetting a small amount of whole blood into a premeasured solution and reading the depth of color in a colorimeter. The companion test to hemoglobin is the hematocrit, also called packed cell volume (PCV). That is a measure of what percentage of the blood is cells as compared to plasma (the liquid part of the blood before it clots). At that time, a hematocrit was done by drawing blood into a tiny glass cylinder, stopping up one end with clay and spinning the small tube in a high powered centrifuge. There was a grid under the tubes that would give you the reading where the liquid ended and the packed cells began. Both were low in this boy. I had stained his slide for the differential and was very disturbed by what I saw under the scope. There were cells which should not have been released from the bone marrow at that early stage. I did not know what cell line they represented but I knew they were not normal. I took the lab report back to the ordering doctor and told him that I did not like the looks of those cells. We sent the slide to the pathologist at the hospital and this unfortunate young man did have leukemia. And he had wanted to play football! It is a lesson on how fragile life can be and how tragedy can strike when we least expect it.

We had brittle diabetics. One lady had given herself too much insulin and was sliding down the door frame of the laboratory when I caught her before she passed out. We had patients with RA (rheumatoid arthritis). At that time the standard treatment was an infusion of gold. Those patients had to have bloodwork before they had their injections to make sure no detrimental side effects were occurring. We got to know those patients very well. We had a doctor as a patient though he was not one of our doctors. Nevertheless, he thought he should have special treatment and would barge in ahead of many fasting patients who had been waiting. Only after we had drawn and tested his blood many times, did we learn that he had Hepatitis B, a contagious disease passed in blood and body fluids. That was in the days before we wore gloves or fluid impermeable lab coats. I did develop the antibodies to that disease, though I never got sick, and I can only believe that I picked it up due to the failure of that doctor to warn us.

We became very familiar with certain patient symptoms. It became something of a game to diagnose mononucleosis by watching how the patient (often an adolescent) plopped into the drawing chair for a blood test. This disease, caused by the Epstein Barr virus, results in extreme fatigue and it is passed around in a school so that, after the first victim, we had a heads up that we would be seeing it again.

I got to see some unusual conditions in our patients. I first saw aplastic anemia in this clinic. The patient had been a radiologist when young and had not been appropriately shielded from the radiation. He was quite old when he came to us and already knew why the production of cells in his bone marrow was depressed. This type of anemia was found in survivors of the atomic bomb in Japan.

We also had a patient with scleroderma. It is a rare condition in which the skin thickens. The skin on his forearms had thickened to some extent but we were still able to do venipunctures. His fingertips were very sclerosed and a fingerstick would probably have been impossible.

We did tests I had not done at the hospital, such as smears for gonorrhea. The bacteria causing that disease, Neisseria gonorrhea, stains gram negative with a gram stain and are little bean-looking organisms that fit together as a pair, facing each other. They are unmistakable and

I got to see the treatment regimen when the nurses would use our heat block to try to warm the penicillin because the injection hurts a lot more if it is cold. There were two big syringes of it, one for each hip and the idea of that was enough to keep me on the straight and narrow forever.

Pinworms were common and we did a lot of scotch tape preps, especially on kids. Pinworms are not life-threatening but they cause itching. The tiny worms come out in the evening and the mother would be instructed to press a piece of clear scotch tape to the area beside the rectum before the child was bathed and put to bed. She would then stick it on to a glass slide we had given her and we would put the slide under the scope. If present, we could see the ova quite clearly or even an adult worm.

I had not done much microbiology at the hospital but my coworker was very helpful and it soon became my favorite of all departments. We were not set up to do anaerobic cultures so they had to be sent out. Anaerobic bacteria live in areas without oxygen, such as in the intestines or in the roots of teeth. Anaerobic conditions must continue during the incubation of anaerobic cultures and we did not have the proper equipment for that. But we had plenty of aerobic cultures. Urines are aways the most common. Many doctors prescribe antibiotics for a first urinary infection without culturing because it is so often E coli and easily treatable but subsequent infections need to be identified and the proper antibiotic ordered.

When we culture, we also do sensitivities to various antibiotics. At that time, we identified the organism after it grew out on media with some simple biochemical tests, then inoculated a special medium with a dilution of the organism and used small disks impregnated with various antibiotics. If the organism grew up to the edges (or even over) the disk, the organism was resistant to that drug and it could not be used. There were calipers to measure the size of the zone around the disk to determine whether the sensitivity of the drug was satisfactory or only moderate.

We did a lot of strep cultures as well. Streptococcus pyogenes (Strep A) is a common infection that can have disastrous sequelae. One of the nurses showed me her method of taking a culture from a patient. She had the patient stick out his tongue, then took a 4×4 piece of sterile gauze, grabbed the tongue firmly and gently pulled it forward. It really opened up the throat so I could see what I was doing with the swab. That is important, since strep creates white areas of infection that should be swabbed for testing.

At that time, many people still went back north in the summer so the lab slowed down. They asked me to substitute for one of the nurses while she was on vacation and subsequently, for one of the secretaries. I was not much of a substitute nurse as I was supposed to find out what drugs the patient was taking. Since I didn't know much about drugs, if they said they were on a "little white heart pill," that is exactly what I wrote down. Probably not very helpful. This was a valuable experience as I got to see the before and after of treatment but, more than that, it gave me a real appreciation for what the nurses and secretaries did every day. Some patients were very needy and it took a lot of patience and understanding to deal with them. I realized it was probably a good thing that I had not become a nurse.

Over time, I got to know the doctors, PAs and nurses as people with their own doubts, personal problems and joys. We were able to see any of our doctors free of charge which was a big plus since I had two young children with the usual ailments. There were parties. My husband wore a full head mask which he had torn and sewn up (poorly) to go to a Halloween party and our resident surgeon, also a guest, told him he should sue for such a bad stitching effort. We were a family. I worked there for five years and there were the expected troubled marriages, divorces and remarriages but, believe me, it was not *General Hospital*. I have never worked any place where real healthcare workers had time for that many affairs.

One of our resident doctors was interested in doing missionary work in what was then British Honduras (now Belize). He brought a young man up to learn basic lab work and the other tech and I trained him. He was bright and willing but he tended to be judgmental. If we had a patient with a venereal disease, he expressed the opinion that they did not deserve treatment. The same attitude was shown to those who used drugs. We really came down on him for this thinking as one of the first things you learn when working in medicine is that it is not your place to judge. You are there to treat, not to criticize.

Interview with the Face of the Lab

Name, shift and duties, how long have you worked in the lab?

My name is Jennifer Troutman. I work day shift in a hospital as a medical laboratory assistant in histology. Histology is a special department of the lab. Histo techs take the tissue that is removed during surgery or other procedures and slice it thinly. They then stain it so the pathologist can examine it under the microscope and decide whether there is cancer or other disease process. We do not do histology onsite in my hospital anymore except for frozen sections. Those are done by the pathologist while the patient is still on the table so that the surgeon can know whether the tissue he has already removed is all of the cancer or whether he needs to take more. For specimens that need to be prepared in the regular histology department, my job is to get them ready and send them out as soon as possible so that the histo techs at our sister hospital can process them.

I have worked in different areas of healthcare. I started out as an EMT up north. Then I did physicals for insurance companies before training as a lab assistant. Lab assistants do phlebotomy, get the samples ready for the techs and other support functions. I have worked in that capacity for twenty-five years. I like to learn new things and have enjoyed working with the doctors and techs to learn more about medical procedures.

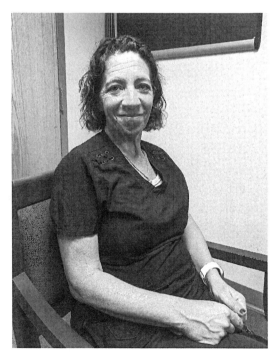

Jennifer Troutman, MLA

What is the biggest challenge for you in your job?

I think ordering the correct option on the computer is my biggest challenge. There are various testing procedures for any specimen and I want to make sure the right one is ordered. I have people to ask if I am unsure and I am not afraid to ask for their help.

Is your job different since Covid? How did it affect you during the epidemic?

I was working as the lab assistant coordinator

during Covid. I didn't collect the patient samples for Covid testing. Mostly, nurses did that but it was up to me and the other assistants to get the samples to the lab for testing. All of us were really swamped. The ambulances were sitting in the parking lot waiting to get in. These were sick patients. If our hospital was full, we had to find another place to send them. We needed to get the results of the Covid testing before we could admit them so it put a lot of pressure on the lab.

Do you feel stressed in your job? If so, do you have some on-the-job support?

I was stressed during Covid. At first, supervisors did not think we needed to wear all of the protective equipment in our job because they didn't think we would be seriously exposed but when lab assistants started getting Covid, they instituted new protocols. We had to wear our ordinary scrubs, surgical scrubs over that and a PPE gown over all. We had to use two sets of gloves and a respirator mask with a paper mask over the respirator. It was a scary time. I did feel supported by my coworkers. We were all in it together.

How does your work affect home life? Do you find it difficult to balance work and the rest of life? How do you handle childcare, if applicable?

I have four adult kids and five stepkids. The youngest is 18 so no more childcare for them but I am also raising three grandchildren, ages 9, 8 and 8. Daycare for them is very expensive. In this job, I don't have to work weekends and that is important because of the kids. My husband works on a ship. He is away for 28 days, then home for 14. It's rough when he's away but, when he is home, he takes over and I get a break.

Do you feel that you are recognized as part of the healthcare team?

Yes. Definitely. I work directly with the pathologists so that's interesting. At first, we were buried in the basement but now, I've been involved with cat scans and ultrasound. I like being visible. You have to find your niche.

Do you feel satisfaction in your work? Are you glad you went into the field?

Yes, definitely. Previously, when I worked as an assistant in the ER, it was too nerve wracking. My training as an EMT and in the ER did prepare me for life saving, though. I had to do the Heimlich maneuver on a grandkid and I performed CPR on a shopper in Home Depot. I even had to use the defibrillator.

Would you recommend young people go into this field? Why or why not? What would you tell them about the field?

Yes. Young people don't seem to know about the lab field when they begin their higher education. Lab assistants are the face of the hospital. If they are drawing blood, they see every patient. Histology techs are in great demand but most people have never heard of the field. We need to get the word out there.

THREE

Moving Up,
Exam After Exam

While working at the clinic, I had continued my studies and I received my AA degree in 1981. That made me eligible to take the test to qualify for the Medical Technologist license. At the time, there were separate exams for each specialty of the lab. I took the tests in hematology, chemistry, serology/immunology and microbiology and passed all four. I did not take the test immunohematology (blood bank) as I didn't feel that I had enough experience in that discipline at the time, though it was added later. An AA degree wasn't enough, however. To be nationally registered as a medical technologist required a four-year degree with specific course requirements and many of the science courses were not offered at night. I decided to get a job that would allow me to take some classes during the daytime. Working in the clinical lab was out because illness does not wait, patients do not stop coming and a tech's presence is required every day. So, I tried my hand at a nonclinical lab.

I worked in the environmental section of a water management district. Many tests required the same skills and the pay was better. We did titrations such as we had used for chloride in my first job. These were to discover whether there had been saltwater intrusion into wells on the coast. We measured dissolved oxygen in water samples from lakes and other bodies of water to monitor pollution. We used probes to measure ammonia levels for the same reason. We also had an atomic absorption spectrophotometer that looked for metallic elements in the water. We had QC charts very similar to those in the clinical lab though the standards did not have to be quite so rigorous. It was an interesting job and I occasionally got to go with one of the biologists to collect samples, but the main advantage was that I could take time off during the day to attend a university close by. I had to make up the time by working later but I felt it was worth it.

My first course was called pre-calculus. It was actually college level algebra and trigonometry. The time was convenient for my schedule, and it was a required course for a biology degree at St. Leo College. I had chosen this private college because of its proximity. I had been driving to Tampa to the University of South Florida, a trip that took hours each way and I didn't have hours to lose. St. Leo did offer a medical technology degree but I had already learned the manual skills that would be included in their intern program. The ASCP (American Society of Clinical Pathologists) was the governing body in charge of making the rules and administering the exams for national registry. Degrees in biology, chemistry or microbiology were acceptable to them so long as enough job experience was authenticated.

Bear in mind that I had not taken any algebra in 25 years and I really struggled but my professor was encouraging. We had access to a tutor, a Cuban lady who had many stories to tell about old Cuba, including one about watching a young Fidel Castro from her upstairs window as he sat at a café table beneath her and laid his machine gun on the tablecloth. Her husband had been considered an enemy of the state and they had been forced to emigrate. Tears of frustration came to my eyes when dealing with homework for that class but I got through it and came out of that course with a B.

They were looking for a supervisor at the environmental lab but that position required a four year degree and I didn't bother to apply. Not only did I not have the degree, I still preferred the clinical lab. Other courses were needed and I wasn't getting any younger. There were some courses I could still take at the community college that St. Leo would accept toward my degree. So, in 1983, I went back to medicine.

This time, it was a much larger clinic with forty doctors and physician assistants. We had new equipment and I went to Dallas to train on the new multi-test chemistry analyzer. This machine was a big step up from using individual cuvettes (test tubes) and running the tests one at a time but it still took two days to get a profile done. It did not have the capacity to run all the analysis on our number of patients in one day so we had to run half on one day and the other half the next. We were still drawing patients and it kept three of us busy doing chemistry, hematology, urinalysis and basic micro. We also had a walk-in clinic next door to the lab and we were often called to help with patients in the walk-in.

There was no hospital on our side of the county at that time and I started calling it the Crawl-In clinic because we got cases that should have gone directly to the hospital. I well remember one Code Blue I was called on to assist because the nurse, an LPN, could not get the IV started and I had to help. Of course, that was not in my job description, but when someone is dying, you don't argue. We did have a defibrillator and we got the patient back but it was a hairy time. Another instance was a GI (gastrointestinal) bleed. When we picked the patient up to transfer him to the gurney for the ambulance, blood ran all over the floor. The work never stopped but I was making the heady amount of $5.00 an hour in 1983.

I was continuing my education when I could get courses that fit my schedule. I enjoyed taking microbiology and wound up doing almost all the micro in our lab. We saw a bigger variety of tests with the larger patient population. I saw sickle cells in patients rather than just the ones we had studied in school. The red cells are indeed sickle shaped when viewed under the microscope, and they tend to clog the blood vessels, the spleen and the joints, resulting in great pain for the patient. It is caused by an abnormal hemoglobin molecule, hemoglobin S, which is not found in normal hemoglobin. The condition only appears if the child gets two copies of the abnormal hemoglobin gene. If a child gets only one copy, he or she will be somewhat anemic but won't have the awful crises seen with sickle cell disease. If a patient has only a single copy of the gene, that condition is called sickle cell trait. It is entirely up to the tech to recognize abnormal cells when doing a differential. The slide will go to the pathologist only if the tech flags that slide for review or if the ordering physician orders a path review directly.

Using a microscope takes practice. One of the first things I learned is that, if we wore mascara, it had to be the waterproof kind. Otherwise, black smudges would start to appear on the oculars, occluding the field. There are normally three objective lenses, ×10, ×40 and ×100. These magnifications are augmented by the 10× magnification of the ocular (eyepiece). The low power (×10) is used to quantify some cells in urine after an aliquot of urine is spun down in a centrifuge and the sediment is mixed and put on a slide with a coverslip. These cells may be epithelial (likely contamination from the skin) or renal and transitional, which could indicate kidney disease. It is important to know the difference. Casts are also enumerated under low power and can be hyaline, which are likely normal, or white or red cell casts, which can indicate infection. Fatty casts can signify kidney disease.

Bacteria are also seen under the scope but bacteria, red cells and white cells are reported using the high power (40×) objective. Other items may be seen under the scope such as yeast cells, spermatozoa and various crystals. There are also lots of what we called UFOs, unidentified floating objects, in some urines. Talcum powder contaminates the urine specimen with shiny circular crystals. When crystals break down, they leave sediment that is just reported out as amorphous or as debris.

The oil immersion (100×) lens is used for blood smears after the thin film of blood has been dried and stained with Wright stain. A small drop of oil is added to the dried and stained slide and this eliminates refraction at this high magnification (1000× including the 10× ocular). Wright stain consists of methylene blue and eosin in an alcohol solution. They used to be separate stains but new solutions mix the two together. The methylene blue stains the nuclei of the white cells blue. If the cells are not stained, the white cells are colorless. This allows us to be able to differentiate the type of cell. Neutrophils or segs (short for polysegmented cells) are usually the most numerous type of white cell. They increase when there is a bacterial infection.

Lymphocytes are mononuclear and there are several kinds. Antibodies are made by lymphocytes and they can live for many years which is why you do not get the same viral infection again if your immune system is normal. Basophils have darkly stained granules. The red (eosin) stain colors the granules in eosinophils which allows the tech to differentiate them from segs. Platelets also stain blue. Red cells stain red and any inclusions in the red cells will take a contrasting stain. Any inclusion in a red cell needs investigation. Certain types of hereditary conditions can cause inclusions in the red cells. Basophilic stippling is seen in abnormalities of hemoglobin or it can indicate lead or other heavy metal ingestion in the patient. An experienced tech will look for all these possibilities and others when perusing a smear.

We had begun to wear scrubs in this lab. They were a great improvement over white uniforms but no color was safe from the chemicals we used. If you wore a dark color, bleach would find it and leave telltale spots. If you wore light colors, the gram stain or Wright stain would make nasty splotches. In a few months, I didn't have a single unmarked scrub set. We did have our short coats but they didn't offer much in the way of protection. This was long before the safety practices instituted later in clinical labs and we definitely had some unsafe practices. Tech Midge tells me that they used carbon tetrachloride whenever they had a stain on their coats or scrubs. They just doused the stain as soon as they saw it and it worked very well but we now know that breathing carbon tetrachloride is hazardous and it is also a possible carcinogen. Some techs smoked in the lab and we thought nothing of drinking our coffee at the bench or snacking. Should we have known better? Yes, but we all have a tendency to do as we see done, especially when we are new to the position.

We still had the privilege of seeing the doctors in the clinic for free but they were busy so, if it was a very simple ailment, our pathologist would sometimes write a prescription for us. My daughter had a sore throat and a positive strep test. Our path wrote a script for penicillin but Eve was upset when I told her. The only pathologist she knew was Quincy of television and she knew he did autopsies. So, when I explained where I had gotten the script, she exclaimed "Oh, Mommy, now you're taking me to the dead people's doctor."

Childcare was an ongoing problem. Though I did not have to work weekends or holidays at the clinic, the summer months when the kids were out of school, were a challenge. My son was now 16 and my daughter was 11. You might think that they were old enough to stay alone but I would get phone calls from home such as "Mom, he's eating all the doughnuts." Or my son, who was driving, would want to go somewhere and I could not leave my daughter alone. My friends and I traded children throughout the summer as most of them worked, too, and it became a scramble to find the one that could take my daughter that particular day. In return, I took theirs on weekends since some still worked in the hospital. I also signed them up for any summer camp that interested them. As a last resort, my daughter went to summer recreation run by the county but she hated it and I suffered the working mother's guilt pangs when I had to insist that she go when she did not want to.

Once I got childcare covered and was at work, I had to put everything else out of my mind. It was critical that the tests we did be accurate. A sugar reported as high when it was actually low, could result in insulin being erroneously given and death could result. One of the most critical tests, the prothrombin time, was common but of great importance. Because bleeding or the opposite, clotting, is so important, testing of the coagulation system must be done, especially in patients who are on an anticoagulant or who have a history of clots. The prothrombin time, abbreviated protime or PT and the APTT (activated partial thromboplastin time) are routinely done prior to any surgery. There are hereditary and acquired bleeding and clotting disorders that could affect bleeding during surgery or make the patient more susceptible to clots afterwards.

Many people take blood thinners because they have had blood clots or heart attacks caused by a clot in the vessel or by plaque which has occluded it. It is imperative to keep watch on the efficacy of blood thinners such as warfarin (coumadin) as an overabundance can result in uncontrolled bleeding or too low a dose could result in another clot. There are 13 factors involved in the clotting of blood. It is one of the most complicated systems that techs must learn. A normal PT is 11–13 sec and a normal APTT is 30–40 sec (Merck, 2022). For patients taking blood thinners the doctor wants to prolong the protime. When I began working in clinics, we used an optical method of obtaining protime results. A small amount of reagent was added to a measured amount of the patient's anticoagulated blood. The tech started a stopwatch as soon as the two mixed, then rocked the tube gently and watched for a clot to form. This method required practice and a sharp eye.

The APTT is prolonged in hemophilia while the protime is normal. There are two types of hemophilia but the most common is caused by a lack of Factor VIII. It is one of the sex-linked diseases, meaning the deficient gene is passed only through the mother on the X chromosome. Under normal circumstances, if a female child gets the faulty X, she will still not develop the disease because she also got a normal X from the father (females get two X's and males get one X from the mother and a Y from the father). If a male child gets the faulty X he will develop hemophilia. It is a sad disease because the child must always be leery of doing anything which might cause him to bleed, limiting childhood activities. If there is a bleed, he must be given Factor VIII along with other treatment. The mother with the faulty X will not necessarily have hemophiliac sons because she has one normal X which she is just as likely to pass on as the defective one. However, she has a fifty-fifty chance of passing the defective gene to a daughter who can then have sons who suffer the disease. There have been very rare instances when a female child developed the disease, usually because one X carried hemophilia and the other was defective or nonfunctional.

There are also hereditary problems with blood clotting and they are not all that uncommon. One young mother I knew did not have any idea she had a condition called Von Willibrand until she gave birth and bled profusely. Another man developed blood clots in his leg and lung and, when tested, was found to have an abnormality in one of the clotting factors. His children needed to be tested along with his siblings. This condition, Factor V Leiden, causes the patient to be ten times more likely to develop clots. They have the condition from birth but it hardly ever causes clots until later adulthood. This man was in his sixties. You can't escape your genes.

Of course, chemistry tests are necessary for diagnosing many abnormal conditions. The most common is blood glucose, which we just call sugar, for diagnosing and monitoring diabetes. Diabetics need to come in for regular blood glucose levels. They may use a glucometer at home but they are often not as accurate as a glucose done in the lab. Also, glucometers must be calibrated. Calibration is common in the lab and requires the running of known standards. New lots of strips required a calibration step back then and I found that many patients did not understand the need for this step and they were not getting accurate results when they performed the test at home. There are many sad glucose stories. When a diabetic patient comes into the ER, the first thing to be decided is whether they are high or low. There are physical signs for both conditions but a stat glucose is always on order. Conditions other than diabetes can affect sugar.

One patient, who had never been diabetic, had an elevated sugar on her profile. A normal fasting glucose should be 70–105 mg/dl (Merck, 2022). Normal values are reconsidered as time goes on and some indicate that the level should be 100 or less. When we investigated this patient's history, we found that she had been taking prednisone and it can elevate blood sugar. Low blood sugar can also be scary. In the clinics we often ran glucose tolerances. A given amount of glucose is given by mouth and the blood is drawn at intervals for several hours to see how that particular patient's body metabolizes it. Some people metabolize quickly and their sugar can drop too low. The usual treatment for that is to eat small protein rich meals more often. Another test is the O'Sullivan test, which is a shorter glucose tolerance and is done between the sixth and seventh month of pregnancy to determine if the mother is subject to gestational diabetes. That can be important as, in addition to all the problems associated with ordinary diabetes, the baby may also get too large.

During my employment in this clinic, circa 1983, a representative from Apple computers brought in a system for us to observe. We were all entranced by the little worm eating the apple and even more entranced when he showed us how we could enter our data (the readings obtained when running controls) and this marvelous machine would draw our control graph for us and figure out the standard deviation. It could also take the readings from our standards and draw our curve. Gone would be the big sheet of log paper. I was hoping the clinic would spring for this invention. They eventually did. This was only the beginning of computer use in the clinical lab. Little did we know how it would affect every facet of medicine.

In microbiology we were using small panels to identify organisms. They consisted of short plastic strips with small individual pockets containing chemicals. When these pockets were inoculated with a suspension from a bacterial culture and incubated, chemical reactions would take place within the pockets depending on the organism introduced. It was certainly a step up from using individual tubes to see color changes brought about by organisms and reading each individually but, in order to see that all was well, it required that known organisms be purchased as quality control and the results must show that the panels identified the organism successfully.

A new test I really hated at this clinic was blood gas analysis. None of us had been trained to do this test as it is usually a function of the Respiratory department, but they had not yet received the required licensing, so they drew arterial blood and we ran it. Of course, levels of oxygen and CO_2 are vitally important, especially in the diagnosis and monitoring of emphysema and COPD (chronic obstructive pulmonary disease) but the method at the time could be frustrating. The machine had a tiny membrane with a very small O ring that had to be stretched over it without even the tiniest wrinkle. I felt like I was all thumbs and really dreaded seeing a blood gas come in.

While I was at this clinic, we had a state inspection. Larger clinic labs such as ours, as well as hospital labs, were required by the state of Florida to be licensed and inspected at intervals. There are many requirements for quality control in the lab. In hematology, controls are preserved suspensions of cells purchased from reputable suppliers for use specifically in the lab. They come in low, normal and high values in order to make sure the cell counters are operating properly at all levels. Chemistry controls come for every analyte and all of these controls in every department must be run at least once daily, and often they are run every shift.

There are controls for coagulation studies such as those described above. In a licensed lab, the results obtained on control values are graphed. Calculations are done and results must come within 2SD (standard deviation) of the mean. This is done for every analyte, and, at that time, we had not yet bought the computer so it was a laborious process. If a result does not come within the required range, the process is examined. It may be a need to recalibrate, a need for new control or even tech error.

An inspector examines control charts first of all. All control values must be within the required range and any outliers researched and noted in an action log. We were very careful to make sure our values were good. He then looked at our procedure manuals. Every test must have a written procedure. They must be up to date and signed by the presiding pathologist. He also looked at our individual licenses to make sure we were compliant with the licensure rules. I was not the supervisor in this lab but I had been asked to work with the inspector. It is a lengthy process and I guess he noticed that I had written many of the procedures and was doing all the micro. He asked me whether I had considered taking the test for supervisor which I had not considered up to this point. He told me that the state was going to change the requirements. At the present time, all that was required to take the exam for supervisor was 90 credit hours of college, including 30 credit hours of science and ten years of experience. If I waited, he said, the state was going to require a four-year degree to be a supervisor. His words were, "You are obviously doing the work. You might as well have the position." I decided right then to continue taking all the science courses I could and to try to get the license before the rules were changed.

Our local community college offered a limited number of science courses. I took them all but was forced to drive to the University of South Florida in Tampa to take genetics as St. Leo did not offer the course that particular semester and I wanted to get those science hours before the state of Florida required even more schooling. I well remember that course in genetics which was given in an auditorium in an abbreviated time period in summer. It was very difficult for me as I was working, too, and still raising a family. In the meantime, I took the HEW exam. This was an exam given by the National Department of Health and Human Services, Public Health Services, Centers for Disease Control. I believe it was an effort by the Federal Government to try to standardize qualifications for laboratory personnel, which varied greatly from state to state. I knew that I could work anywhere in the USA if I passed the HEW test while my licensure was only good for Florida. It still was not as good as national registry with the ASCP, which was the pinnacle of laboratory certification but that required a four-year degree which seemed a long way off at the time. I did pass the HEW and felt that certification was another tool on my belt.

Eventually, I obtained all the credit hours necessary and was approved to take the exams that would allow me to work as a supervisor in a Florida lab. There was an exam for each specialty plus a management exam. I passed them all and obtained my supervisor's license in 1985.

Changes had taken place in the clinic. A new person had been brought in to be in charge and his wife was a medical technologist. They fired the person who had been the manager and put the wife in charge of the lab. I would have had no problem with this move if she had actually worked but the truth was, we very seldom saw her. The problem for me was that it was my supervisor's license hanging on the wall but I was not the supervisor. It was not a comfortable situation and I left there not long after receiving the license.

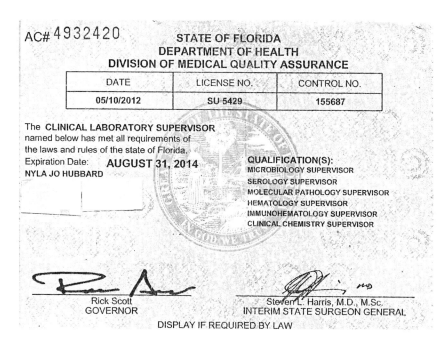

My most recent license before I retired.

FOUR

Specialty Patients: Oncology/Hematology

For two years, I did not work in the lab. My husband had developed some property we owned. I took the course and got a real estate license, then sold the lots and dealt with contracts and closings. It wasn't long before I missed the lab, however. Real estate might have paid better but science and medicine were what I loved and I tried to do both by taking a parttime position with a hematology/oncology clinic nearby.

The tests we did were very simple, mostly CBCs to make sure the chemo being given was not depressing the bone marrow too much. If the patient's white cell level got too low, they would be susceptible to infection. If that happened, or if they got too anemic, the chemo could not be given, so blood was drawn before they even saw the doctor.

Blood drawing could be challenging because many of these patients had been drawn many times and had experienced many IVs and their veins were scarred and hard to find. I did enjoy getting to know the patients individually. There were also many conditions I had not seen before. I remember one patient with hemochromatosis. This condition can be either hereditary or acquired but the hereditary form is more common (Mayo, Mayo Clinic, 1998–2022). It results in an overload of iron. The heredity is similar to that of the Rh factor so that a child must inherit a gene for the condition from both parents. Some people who have the homozygous (two of the same gene) heredity never have symptoms and, in any case, the condition seldom expresses itself before middle age. Women with the condition develop it later in life than men do. The excess iron can cause pain in the joints and in severe cases, cirrhosis or liver failure. The acquired form can come about from too many blood transfusions as might be given for a hemophiliac or from long-term alcoholism. The patient in this clinic was an alcoholic and the main symptom I remember were his blue fingertips. They were very noticeable.

After I drew and ran the blood through my cell counter, some patients went on to radiation. Our radiation techs were a couple from Jamaica. They were always very professional, the male of the pair wearing a long white well starched coat. I liked hearing their lovely, melodic accents and the patients loved them.

I was asked to help with bone marrow collection. Both white and red cells as well as megakaryocytes, the progenitors of platelets, are formed in the bone marrow. Bone marrow taps are usually done from the hip. It is necessary to look at the cells developing in the bone marrow to determine whether a particular condition is the result of inadequacy in the bone marrow itself because it is making too many, too few or nonfunctional cells or whether there is destruction of cells after they leave the bone marrow. Bone marrow is comprised of stem cells. There are two kinds. Myeloid stem cells develop into red cells, neutrophilic white cells, eosinophils and basophils. They can also develop into megakaryocytes which will fragment before going into the circulating blood as platelets. The myeloid cells which are the parents are called myeloblasts.

The other kind of stem cell is the lymphoid stem cell. That cell will go either into the lymph nodes or into the thymus. The thymus is active in childhood but decreases in size as people age. This gland is located behind the breastbone. It is thought that the ancient Greeks named it thymus because they thought it bore a resemblance to thyme, a cooking herb (Eldridge, 2022). One purpose of the thymus is to turn out T cell lymphocytes, a cell which you will hear more about as we talk about AIDS. Sometimes, these blasts can be seen in the peripheral (circulating) blood in leukemias and other blood dyscrasias. It is up to the tech viewing the slide to call attention to these precursor cells so that the slide can be examined by the hematologist or the pathologist.

I well remember one patient who was having a bone marrow aspiration. He asked to hold my hand and that was fine though he was actually gripping my wrist. The doctor numbed the area of the hip where the needle would be inserted and, before he could even insert the needle, the patient stiffened and moaned. More numbing agent was used but the entire procedure seemed to be a terrible ordeal for the patient and my wrist was actually bruised from his grip. When we were outside the room, I asked the doctor why this procedure seemed to have generated so much more pain than was usual. The doctor, with utmost understanding, said that everyone had a level of pain tolerance and it wasn't the patient's fault if his was low.

I mentioned having seen a patient in my first job who had multiple myeloma. We will call her Mildred. She was in excruciating pain. Multiple myeloma is a cancer of the blood in which B lymphocytes are activated and start turning out antibodies. That is the function of B lymphocytes. However, these antibodies are not normal and they do not protect. They multiply in the bone marrow and spill out into the circulating blood. Then a new kind of cell is seen on the smear called a plasmacyte. It is an eyeball shaped cell and is always cause for alert though a few are not necessarily abnormal. In multiple myeloma, special proteins build up in the blood and spill out into the urine. We use a method called immunoelectrophoresis to separate the proteins. The Bence-Jones protein is indicative of multiple myeloma. The proliferation of cells in the bone marrow can cause bone pain, which is one of the worst. I will never forget Mildred and her suffering. I think it is a shame that techs seldom get out on the floor anymore. Seeing the patient makes that tube of blood you are handling much more personal.

We had patients with platelet abnormalities. Some had too many, a condition called thrombocythemia since the proper name for a platelet is thrombocyte. You would think that these patients would clot more easily and they can, but they can also bleed because the platelets don't function properly. When looking at the smear, the tech will see not only too many platelets but they can also be large or clumped together. The opposite is the patient with thrombocytopenia, too few platelets. This can be the result of some drug therapy or it can result from an antibody which has formed for an unknown reason and that antibody attacks the body's own platelets. We often had to do platelet transfusions for this condition but the antibody would attack the new platelets, too. It was a difficult condition to treat.

We had one patient with polycythemia vera, a condition in which they have too many white cells, too many red cells and too many platelets, stemming from overproduction in the bone marrow. Patients report light-headedness or headache due to the blood being too thick. The treatment was therapeutic phlebotomy.

Often, patients would come in with their spouse. In one case the wife had cancer and it had been a slog for her as it was well advanced and the treatment regimen was long. Her husband came in as a patient once.

He had CLL (chronic lymphocytic leukemia), a type of blood cancer fairly common in older people and one which may not necessarily lead to death. I thought he always looked tired and possibly anemic and those are symptoms of the disease. He always expressed concern only for his wife. We were very sad to hear that he had died suddenly. He was a lovely person and now who would care for the remaining and very ill wife? It was just one example of how important it is to care for the caregiver.

Of course, there were many cancer patients. One patient had liver cancer and was the color of a pumpkin. Jaundice is caused by the buildup of bilirubin. Most bilirubin comes from the end products of red cells which only live three to four months before they are broken down by phagocytic cells in the spleen due to wear and tear. The bilirubin is then normally processed by the liver and excreted in the stool which gives feces their normal brown color. When it can't be excreted, as when the liver is diseased, bilirubin builds up in the blood and turns the skin and the whites of the eyes yellow. This patient seemed so unwell when I left that clinic that I thought he was near death but, when I went back at Christmas time to leave some cookies, there was an ornament that he had made for me with my name on it. The staff said he was still doing OK.

I thought, when I took the job, that it would be sad because we would be losing so many patients but I was surprised at how long our doctors could keep people going with a decent quality of life. These doctors were of Indian descent and Hindu religion but it was obvious that it is not only the Christion ethic to practice kindness and generosity. Chemo drugs are usually expensive and some patients could not pay but I never knew of a patient who was refused care at this clinic because of money. Some debt must have been carried for years or just written off.

Statistics Show That New Methods of Detection and Therapy Are Prolonging or Saving the Lives of Cancer Victims (NIH, 2022)

Dr. Lisa Coussens, MD, said "that part of the credit goes to an investment in research—both for treatments and for understanding the disease."

"Targeted therapies, immunotherapy, and other new approaches being applied clinically all stem from fundamental discoveries in basic science" (Hassan, 2022).

These new therapies are the result of new molecular testing done in the clinical lab such as those mentioned in Chapter Twelve of this book.

FIVE

Education:
In the Lab and
In the Classroom

My children were getting older and I longed to get back to the hospital with its greater variety. I also was determined to get that four-year degree. The Clinical Laboratory Information Act, better known as CLIA, had been passed in 1988. This act attempted to standardize quality control and staffing in the clinical lab. Despite having the Florida supervisor's license and HEW certification, I learned that I could not be a Medicare-approved supervisor at that time without a baccalaureate degree. The lack of that degree would mean that I could never be in charge of a larger lab that accepted Medicare, which almost all labs do. I learned that St. Leo College (now University), where I had taken my precalculus course, would accept all of my credits from prior colleges. This was important because most universities accept only 60 credit hours and I had racked up more than that. I was also able to take the CLEP (College Level Placement Exams) tests in several subjects which saved money. In addition, though the private tuition was higher than at a state university; once you paid for twelve credit hours, any more courses were free.

Because the science courses and their labs were all given in the daytime, I took a job in a hospital working second shift, 2:30 until 11 p.m. on the weekends. It is rare that a tech new to the hospital will get a coveted daytime shift. Those positions are usually earned by long employment. My youngest was an older teen but off shifts are tough for a mother with schoolage children as it takes you away from your kids during the only hours when they are out of school and awake. But many start on second or third shift as they have no choice but to take what they can get and wait for an opening on day shift. Other techs choose second shift or night shift because of the shift differential. It was a 10 percent bonus above my hourly rate for second shift and 15 percent above for night shift when I began in the hospital.

Tech friends tell me of creative shifts used during the 1980s. Judy worked what was called a straight 40 hour shift. There were supposed to be two techs who would split the duties for 40 hours, taking turns sleeping during slow periods. One weekend Judy walked into the lab to find that she was to be the only tech on for 40 hours. It was a county hospital which was always cash strapped and the powers that be had decided they could do with just one tech. Judy was worried but thought she might be able to sleep at some time during lulls. It was not to be. There were accidents, heart attacks and lots of babies being born. Judy did not sleep for forty hours. The decision to expect her to work alone was short-sighted to say the least. No one's brain works well after that many hours of sleep deprivation and no one can be expected to be alert and have the proper concentration to assure good patient care under those circumstances. She complained and they did get a phlebotomist to draw the morning bloods but would not hire another tech to share the load in the lab. She stayed just long enough to find another job before she escaped and I hope the management of that hospital learned a lesson.

Another tech tells me about a weekend she was working alone in another county hospital and victims of a massive automobile accident came in. Elaine was called to the ER to draw blood on those patients and saw orders for type and cross for transfusion on every chart. It would have been impossible to crossmatch that many people in under an hour at best. She called the doctor and he said he would tell her which patients were most in need and she could do them first. It was great that she had a doctor who would work with her but it is another example of why the work of techs is so stressful. We are always aware of how critical our work is but, when you have multiple stats, you are left wondering which stat is the "stat-est."

County hospitals have always struggled. Of course, there is the matter of dividing up tax revenue among all the various needs and most county commissioners could not really be expected to understand the running of a hospital. Enough resources are seldom allocated to the county hospital. Bob tells me of a weekend during the 1970s when he worked alone in a county hospital. There should have been two techs but one called in and he had no response from his supervisor. It was bad enough to try to do the job of two people but then he ran out of reagent for the chemistry analyzer. With no other recourse, he called a nearby hospital which was not even in the same system but the tech there loaned him the reagent. The tech probably did not have permission to loan to an outside lab but techs try to support techs. Today, hundreds of rural hospitals are in danger of closing because they can't collect enough in fees to stay open (Thompson, 2023). Though Medicaid does not pay well, it pays something if the patient qualifies. The website https://www.benefits.gov/benefit/1625 lists the requirements for receiving Florida Medicaid.

> To be eligible for Florida Medicaid, you must be a resident of the state of Florida, a U.S. national, citizen, permanent resident, or legal alien, in need of health care/insurance assistance, whose financial situation would be characterized as low income or very low income. You must also be one of the following: • Pregnant, or • Be responsible for a child 18 years of age or younger, or • Blind, or • Have a disability or a family member in your household with a disability, or • Be 65 years of age or older."

In addition, according to the same website, a family of four cannot have an income of more than $39,900 to qualify for Medicaid in Florida. If the family income is even slightly more than that, they do not qualify and if their jobs do not offer health insurance, they will likely be handed a bill which they cannot pay.

I never worked anywhere that I was exposed to killer shifts alone but work could still be stressful. Weekends are always more lightly staffed as everyone wants some weekends off. Techs in hospitals are usually required to work every second or third weekend, depending on staffing. Theoretically, doctors are not seeing and admitting patients on weekends. However, the ER never stops on the weekends so there were many stats and fewer techs to run them. Added to that, at the time I worked at this hospital, the state required that every report be examined and initialed by a medical technologist before going out. On many weekends, the other two techs were technicians and I was the only med tech on. There were three of us to staff hematology, chemistry and blood bank and I had to peruse every report. My name was Jo Jones at the time and my supervisor laughed when he told me how many "flying JJ's" he had seen on the lab reports going out. We were also expected to set up any micro cultures and that was a time-consuming activity that wound up being done at the end of the shift. This was not a good system since it meant the cultures did not have the same time to grow that they would have if they had been set up as soon as the specimens came in. This was my first experience in a for-profit hospital and we did the best we could.

Lab analyzers had advanced greatly by 1988 and could run whole panels on one tube of blood. This was certainly easier and faster than the old way but the volume of tests had also increased and we had to learn to keep these monster machines running. It was kind of like having a child. They had to be fed with reagents. Their waste had to be emptied and one had to be aware of any alerts from the machine telling you it needed something, which it did by emitting a very importunate beeping. It was our joke to say, "Hey, Carol, your baby's crying."

More kinds of tests had been invented and this was the era of the lipid profile since cholesterol had become the watchword of the day. It was a big shift in thinking as, when I began training in 1968, a cholesterol of 300 was considered normal in an older woman. Now, suddenly, everyone was supposed to have a total cholesterol of 200 or less. We were also running HDLs (high density lipoprotein) which is the good cholesterol. We included triglycerides as part of the profile and a calculated LDL (low density lipoprotein), the "bad" cholesterol.

Of course, there is money to be made in medicine as with anything else and, back then, there were few laws about doctors having a vested interest in the labs to which they sent patients. More tests meant more profit for them. I always wondered how many tests we did that were profit driven. The Stark Law, which came in 1989 made it illegal for physicians to send patients to labs or other entities in which they had a financial interest without informing the patients.

Another factor that drives up the cost of medicine in general is the ever-present threat of lawsuit. Emergency Room patients, in particular, get more tests than might be necessary due to the possibility that some lawyer, in the future, might ask in hindsight, "Why didn't you run a CBC?," even when the patient came there with a sprained ankle. When I see every other billboard on the highway advertising personal injury lawyers, I think about the cost of medical care going up with every judgment, whether justified or not.

I also wondered about the humanity of continuing to test patients who were beyond help. As healthcare workers, we are trained to preserve life at all costs. The philosophy relieves us of the decision as to when to stop but it is not always best for the patient. Years ago, I was asked to draw a patient in ICU who was so near death that her blood pressure was far below normal. I tried twice to get blood without success. An ICU nurse came over, looked at the patient and said, "I don't know why this test was ordered. It can't help her." I said that I really hated to stick the patient again under the circumstances and the nurse suggested I just write "unable to obtain" on the order. We looked at each other over the form of this moribund patient and I did as she suggested. It was the only humane thing to do.

There was something of a scandal while I worked at this for-profit hospital. I knew that we took the tube off the smaller analyzer which was used to run a Chem 7, the basic tests, and then put the same tube on the larger analyzer that ran the more extensive profiles. It always seemed like double dipping to me because the larger analyzer ran the same Chem 7 tests again as part of the larger profile. Suddenly, word came down from the Feds that labs were running and charging for the lipid profiles without express orders for them from the doctors. They were also charging Medicare twice for the same tests on the same blood as I had seen. Fines were levied and the stock of this company, as well as that of other companies, took a precipitous plunge. One tech, who had worked there for many years, had to cancel her retirement plans because she had been counting on that stock to finance her retirement. All of us who had 401K plans invested in the company stock took a big hit. People were angry and someone put up two pictures in the lab bathroom. One pic was of a bald terrorist with his hard, flinty eyes and the other was of the CEO of the hospital chain at the time, also bald with the same look. This man later became a big name in Florida but I doubt that he was popular with staff at this hospital. Of course, there are many fine doctors, nurses and technical staff working in for-profit hospitals. Just because I don't like the system doesn't mean that the personnel won't give good care.

The weekend shifts along with responsibility at home and managing the homework added up to a lot of stress but I was finally wearing that long white coat, with my name on it, and I was eager as I rotated between departments, including blood bank. I have never been a blood bank specialist and I never did get into the more esoteric tests involved in blood bank but there were nights when it took two of us to handle emergency transfusions. I recall one night when I was still sitting in the blood bank at 1 a.m. because we had a threatened aneurism and the patient had a known antibody. This meant that we had to check multiple units of donor blood in order to find enough units that did not contain the corresponding antigen which would have resulted in a transfusion reaction in the patient. Many nights I went out to the parking lot at the end of my shift and just sat quietly for a few minutes in my car, adjusting to the silence and decompressing before driving home.

We ran Vitamin B12 (proper name cobalamin) levels by radioimmune assay back then and we were required to wear a monitor badge to make sure we weren't getting too many rads. Vitamin B12 is very important in the body as it is necessary for the production of RNA and DNA and is also involved in creating the myelin sheath around the spinal cord (Viatcheslav, 2014). We often saw the indirect effect of low B12 in hematology. There is a condition called pernicious anemia caused, not by low intake of B12, but rather by the lack of intrinsic factor, a substance made in the stomach lining which allows the absorption of the vitamin. The red cells become very large and are called macrocytes (Hole, 1978). This used to be common in older people but is seen less often now.

This was a tough period in my life as I had finished my first course at St. Leo, organic chem, with a B+ and was encouraged to really dive in and get this degree done. So I foolishly signed up for organic chem ii, invertebrate zoo, cell physiology and calculus all in the same semester. It was a killer schedule. In addition, my marriage, which had never been good, was in trouble. My then husband had never finished high school and he did not like it that I was getting a higher education. He also made it hard financially as his permission was needed for me to get grants or student loans and he would not agree to sign the papers. So I had to work enough to pay the tuition myself. I still had a teenager at home and I knew the situation was hard on her as well as on me.

I wasn't about to drop courses once I had signed up so I took a second job at a second hospital in order to cover the cost of college. I often worked weekend day shift at one hospital and left there to begin a second shift at the other. The population of our area was booming and techs were in demand. I was paid more at the second hospital and, because the first one did not want to lose me, I got an instant $5 an hour raise. I was now making $12 an hour in 1989. I felt that I was progressing but at what cost? It is one of my regrets that I was not able to spend more time with my daughter during those years but I felt that I was forced into it. And who among us does not have regrets?

At the second hospital, I made some great friends who have stayed with me through the years and, because it was small, I got to know some of the nurses and other personnel who came in to get blood for transfusion or to check on results. The smaller hospital had a maternity wing. I had not worked in a place with OB (obstetrics) in a long time. The chimes we heard over the intercom had to be explained. "Rock a Bye Baby" played for all to hear when a child was born. A second rendition quickly following indicated twins. It was a nice change as OB is considered the happy wing of the hospital but it meant I would be running new tests. One of the tests unfamiliar to me was the fern test. The nurse would swab the cervix of the expectant mother and put a small amount of the fluid on a slide with a cover slip. We would then watch to see if it formed a fern-like arrangement under the scope. If it did, it showed the doctor that amniotic fluid was leaking. That might indicate premature delivery or just that labor was about to start.

Another OB story etched in my mind was of the young woman who lived in St. Petersburg, Florida, but was visiting in our area when she began having difficulty. The doctor in the ER could not find a heartbeat and it was determined that her fetus had died in the womb. This precipitated a condition called DIC (disseminated intravascular coagulation). The dead fetus had triggered a reaction in her body which was causing small clots in her vessels. Because her clotting factors were all being used up in this process, she was bleeding profusely. We were called upon to do stat testing for protime and APTT as well as the special tests called fibrin degradation products and D-dimer. I felt sorry for this poor girl who had lost her baby and was suffering this grave reaction as well. She did survive, however, and I hope she went on to have a healthy child sometime in the future.

Tech Debbie tells me a funny story from her OB days. A new mother was asked what she was going to name her newborn son. She replied that she had taken inspiration from the sign outside her hospital room door. That sign said " No Smoking" so she had decided to name him Nosmo. Debbie never learned if she did, in fact, lay that on the child but it was a novel idea.

I did blood bank at the second hospital. Genetics play a big part in Blood Bank. It is called immunohematology, because of the immune reactions that can result when two bloods mix. Many antigens are hereditary. Antigens A and B were discovered by an Austrian immunologist and pathologist named Karl Landsteiner. Until his discovery, direct transfusion had been tried by hooking up donor and recipient directly and running the blood from one to the other. Sometimes this went well and sometimes the recipient had a major reaction and some died. It was not understood why until Landsteiner identified the A and B antigens on the red cells. He was awarded the Nobel prize in Physiology and Medicine in 1930. The fact that some cells have both A and B was discovered the next year (Britannica, 2022). Blood group heredity follows the rules laid down by Gregory Mendel centuries ago when he worked with peas. Every person has two genes for blood group, one from each parent. The two genes are your genotype. If one of your genes is an A or a B and the other is an O, you will group as an A or a B because the A or B antigen is always dominant. This is your phenotype. The O gene you have from your other parent is called a recessive gene. You can pass either of those two genes on to your children. If the other parent of your child also has a recessive O, you may have a group O child though each of you groups as an A or a B. We call the two genes your genotype. A mother who is AO with a husband who is BO can have an O child, an A child, a B child or an AB child. Though O is often recessive, it is still the most common blood group in general.

Blood banks stock several units of each group and type of blood, with more units of the most common groups. Each unit is good for only a specified period of time and, because we don't want the units to be wasted, there is a system for sending units that might outdate to a busier hospital where they are more likely to be used. The system requires constant surveillance and rotation of units. Every blood bank always has at least a few O negative units on hand. One night we had a lady brought in by ambulance who had been hit by a car as she walked across the street with her groceries. It was a very foggy night and our helicopter service could not fly so we couldn't send her to a larger tertiary care hospital as we normally would have done. I went down to the ER to collect samples. The ER crew had her in an inflatable pressure suit which is blown up with air in an effort to stop bleeding but I still saw the blood running out the leg holes of the suit. The other tech and I threw group O Rh negative blood in a cooler and brought it to the ER as there was no time to crossmatch. O neg blood can be given to anyone as the O is actually a zero. The red cells in O type blood do not have any A or B antigens coating them as A or B or AB blood does, so zero antigens. We all did our best and so did the ER staff but the lady still died and it was sad to see the Kash and Karry bag sitting on the chair in the ER when she was gone.

Another night in Blood Bank is etched in my mind. A nurse came running into the lab telling us that they needed a group and type stat. She said they had a young man in the ER who was bleeding so profusely from the stomach that the blood was running down the drains in the floor. They had already drawn blood and I immediately started in on trying to get a group and type, the first step in any crossmatch. When ascertaining blood groups, we use an antibody suspension purchased for that purpose. The cells of Group A blood are coated with the A antigen. If you mix a suspension of that blood with the A antibody in a small tube and spin it down, agglutination will occur in the tube. We watch for it carefully by shaking the tube gently over a magnifying mirror. The same happens with B cells and the B antibody solution and in AB blood both A and B will agglutinate. With O blood there will be no agglutination as there is no antigen on the O red cells. The same method is used for Rh typing.

When I examined the tubes after spinning, I could not believe my eyes. Everything agglutinated, A, B and Rh. Of course, that would be expected in an AB Rh positive person but we also ran a negative control using the patient blood that should never agglutinate. In this case, it agglutinated, too. There was strong agglutination in every tube. I was flummoxed. I made new suspensions with the same result. I called the ER and explained the situation. The nurse said that they had given an injection of Vitamin K just before drawing the blood sample. I called a Blood Bank specialist whom I knew and we could only conclude that might be the problem. They transfused with O neg until a proper crossmatch could be done. These are the nights when you question yourself, your training and whether you should be in this business at all.

I had graduated from community college with a GPA of 4.0 and I guess I thought I could handle anything. But organic chem II was a bear, calculus was challenging to say the least and cell physiology and invertebrate zoo required massive memorization. I did enjoy invertebrate zoo as my professor had specialized in malaria and we studied it extensively. I will tell later how this helped me when I did a Doctors Without Borders mission in Africa but I also saw malaria twice in ER patients who had been traveling.

Steady A's were no more but I got through it and signed up for four more courses that fall including physics.

I had to take my student hat off and put my tech hat on when I got to the hospital on the weekends. I think any tech will tell you that the most stressful time is when a machine goes down. My cell counter stopped giving me results during a very busy time one second shift. This could be caused by a small clot that formed in the tube during a difficult draw or because the phlebotomist did not rock the tube to mix it with the anticoagulant after drawing. We had procedures for cleaning and restarting the machine but the phone rang constantly and we had no secretary on second shift weekends. The nurse was pushing me unmercifully for results. After the fifth call, I finally told her, "It's just me here. I can get this machine up and run your test or I can continue to answer the phone while the machine sits there. Which would you rather I did?" I thought I would get into trouble for that remark but I guess she finally realized that I was doing the best I could. Nights like that were not good for a tech's blood pressure.

A survey of 4613 laboratory professionals was reported in *Lab Pulse.* The survey found that 53.4 percent of laboratory workers reported feelings of high stress at some time during their work life. A stunning 85.3 percent reported experiencing burnout at some point. Despite these statistics, most lab personnel still reported high job satisfaction in their careers (Hayes, 2020). This sums up my own feelings in situations where I was unable to get the work out through no fault of my own. I loved the work but constantly being under the gun with no immediate power to change the situation could give you ulcers. That is one reason I am calling us the hidden heroes of medicine. If a nurse is overwhelmed and cries on the floor, people see it. The only crying I ever saw in the lab was restricted to the bathroom and only the streaks on her cheeks when she came out gave her away.

As I've said, hospital techs work weekends and holidays. There were no exceptions at any of the hospitals where I worked. Even if you had been there thirty years (and some techs had been) you still pulled every other or every third weekend and half of the holidays every year. If you worked Christmas this year and were off Thanksgiving, you got Christmas off next year and you worked Thanksgiving plus at least two other holidays. Because I was a PRN (as needed) at both hospitals at the time, rather than a fulltime tech, I was not on the rotation for holidays but I did work one memorable Christmas Eve at the smaller hospital.

I was on with the lab supervisor who was a great guy and not afraid to work the bench when techs wanted off. Our cell counter went down, not a clot, not a belt, something worse. Christmas Eve is notorious for traffic accidents and we did not have time to do manual counts. George called the hotline and they told him what to do. We pulled a circuit board from the innards of the instrument and he popped one component off while I rummaged through the tool box for another just like it. They all looked basically alike but I had to find the correct one with the tiny multidigit part number. Thankfully, it was there and he managed to get it seated on the board and back into the machine. All was a go after that but there is always a worry that it won't work in that kind of situation. We were always careful to reorder when we used a part but one can never be sure until the part is in your hand and the machine is running again. I was tired and, when I finally got out to my car that night, the windshield was coated with ice. It is not something we often see in Florida, and I had no ice scraper. I finally used the side of my nail file to clear the ice so I could see to drive home.

Computers had not yet made paper lab slips obsolete. Our analyzers used computers but there was still no laboratory system that sent results directly to the floor. We used runners to get the results to the proper place. Even on second shift with fewer techs, the lab is not quiet. At any given time, the phone is ringing, the machines (several of them) are beeping and timers are going off. It creates a stress that you are not consciously aware you have. Hospitals always provide coffee free of charge as they want to keep you going. They don't bother with cream or sugar. If you want them, you go to the dining room.

I find myself still eating much too rapidly today even though the need for it is long over. For too many years, it was take a bite and put a tube on, take another bite and take the tube off. Very seldom did we have an uninterrupted meal. I noticed, at the larger hospital, that we all seemed to consume a lot of sugar. There were often sweets someone had brought in or from a vending machine. When we finally had a moment, we would find ourselves stuffing our mouths with sugar and washing it down with coffee, a reaction no doubt to the adrenaline rush.

We still drew patients at this hospital and the first job on my shift would be to collect specimens. I was somewhat nervous when I had to draw in the psych unit. The outside doors locked behind you. The nurses were all within a glassed-in area off limits and it was just me and the patients. One time, we had a patient just coming off a drug overdose. She was combative and I had to ask for help. It took four people to hold her down while I drew one tube of blood.

During breaks in the school calendar, I worked some day shifts and got to know the day shift techs. We were a diverse bunch as many hospital labs tend to be because training in the lab is similar in other countries. We had Filipinos, Koreans and Puerto Ricans as well as techs from all over the United States. It was fun to learn about their cultures and they sometimes brought in food. I remember perogies from the Polish woman and homemade spring rolls from the Korean tech. I also worked with a gay man who was having major trouble in his love life. One evening shift, he had his call to his roommate on constant redial as he suspected him of infidelity. It was the first time I came to realize that love is love and gay people hurt, too, when it goes bad. Perhaps his partner really was unfaithful. Later, when he tried to donate blood, which was being tested for the HIV virus by this time, he learned he was positive. AIDS was fairly new and not well understood. Some techs didn't even want to use the bathroom after Bill even though we had been told it was not transmissible that way. I learned later that the virus developed into AIDS and Bill died. It was a loss to us and to the lab as he was always willing to help and was very good with machinery.

My last semester at St. Leo went by in a blur. I went through a divorce and my daughter left for college. I struggled through physics II but loved botany. Though, I was getting a biology degree, St. Leo had the courseload geared to premed as many of our graduates would be going into medical, dental, veterinary school or to the lab. I think the botany course was their nod to making it truly bio. My professor for botany was a Catholic priest. I was raised Quaker so he was the first priest I had come to know. He was white but from Jamaica and had that lovely singsong accent. He was an excellent teacher and I came to realize how similar plants are to us. Indeed, my stepson, who has a master's degree in botany, calls plants "slow moving animals." I was particularly entranced by the chloroplasts busily moving around inside the plant cell under the microscope. Father Damien told us the theory that chloroplasts were once free living organisms but were hijacked into becoming part of the plant cell. He said there was also a theory that the mitochondria in our cells, which make the proteins our lives depend on, were also once free-living beings. We owe our lives to these little organelles as we would not survive without plants and proteins.

I finally graduated in 1990. It was a centennial year for St. Leo as it had been a school for 100 years. At first, I had no intention of doing the cap and gown thing but, when I was informed that I would have to pay a fixed amount for the graduation whether I participated or not, I decided I would "walk." There was also a luncheon and, as part of my graduation package, I was given three tickets for the luncheon. There was little decision to be made as to who would be eating it, as my daughter was away at college out of state and immersed in her own final exams. That left my son and my parents. Simple. I did send announcements to my brother and my sister.

I admit to consternation when my sister called and told me how much she wanted to see me walk. She said she had not taken part in her own graduation ceremony and she felt it would give her vicarious satisfaction to watch me. Oh, well, I thought, I'll just have to buy one extra ticket.

My mother was delighted to hear that my sister was coming for graduation. However, she did add, in that sweetly chiding way she had, "Don't you think you should ask your brother and his wife now that you have asked your sister?"

"But, Mom," I said, "Clay has a wife and a child still at home. That would be two more tickets." "Well," she said, "maybe he won't be TOO hurt if you don't ask them."

A classmate saved me from the pangs of guilt. He had three luncheon tickets that he wouldn't be using and which he allowed me to purchase. It was now going to require two cars to get everyone to the ceremony but it was doable. I called and left a message at my brother's house, extending the invitation. His wife called back that evening and left a message on my answering machine. She and her husband and daughter were looking forward to it and, also, their grown daughter would accompany them with her baby. As I trudged across campus for yet another ticket, I could only hope that a ticket would not be required for the baby.

My son arrived from South Florida quite late the night before commencement, late enough for me to worry that he wasn't coming. I was holding up well, though. I was at the finish line and I felt buoyant enough to hide my dismay as I explained to my son, that " when one receives an engraved invitation, occasions of that sort usually require Bass Pro T-shirt."

The big day arrived. The powers that be had decided that all regular graduates would be required to attend Baccalaureate Mass. Until this time, I had hardly been aware that I was attending a Catholic College. Imagine, if you can, a Quaker girl, never exposed to a full-fledged religious production of any kind, now expected to rise and fall at the appropriate moments. It was all so foreign. And I never did figure out the reason for the smokers.

We progressed to the pre-commencement lunch. It really was fun to have my family around, lots of family. And, since this was the 100th anniversary for the college, they had gone all out, with the number 100 in an ice sculpture on the table. People remarked on the excellent quality of the food. My mother remarked that I must have really enjoyed eating lunch at this cafeteria every day. My friend, a fellow student, and I looked at each other and snickered. This food was a very far cry from the watery soup we were used to eating.

Lunch over, we were organized and seated for the commencement address. Does anyone remember what is said at their commencement? It was a blur to me and then it was time to walk. My row rose to their feet. I glanced behind to the rear of the auditorium. A baby was crying and I worried that all this waiting was too much for my little great-niece. As it happened, the little one was sleeping but I did hear from that section, in a bellow only a six foot four, 240 pound son could muster, "Way to go, Ma." I guess he was used to football games.

At last, it was my turn. I stood at the foot of the stairs and looked around. The science instructors were grouped in the first row, looking decidedly bored. They had probably seen so many commencements. My name was called and I mounted the steps. My glance stole to my professors, all of them so well known to me and alternately hated and loved. At the same time, they recognized me. My precalculus and calculus teacher, who had allowed me, as a hardship case to take the original course without the usual prerequisites, leaned forward and smiled widely. My chemistry prof and the tough guy invertebrate zoo and physiology teacher also perked up and were applauding me.

I had done it. Yes, I was 45 and it had taken me 17 years to get a Baccalaureate degree but I was satisfied. I had persevered.

Interview with a Recent Tech (2023)

Please tell us your name, shift and duties.

My name is Eric Linney. I received my ASCP certification in December of 2019 and my Florida medical technologist (also called clinical laboratory scientist) license in January of 2020 just before Covid became really well established. I had already completed a Baccalaureate degree in biology but I needed a way to use it. I discovered a way to do that by enrolling in a partnership program between a local college and a hospital consortium. The hospital group paid for my training as I worked as an LMA, a laboratory medical assistant. This allowed me to work in the lab, not as a technologist but as a phlebotomist and processor, on Saturday and Sunday while I took courses Monday through Friday. In order to act as an LMA, I performed 100 "sticks" (phlebotomies) so I did have patient contact during that time. I later worked as a processor and as an assistant in chemistry and hematology but did not work as a phlebotomist during this time. After I completed my training and got my license, I worked in the main lab for a year until an opening came up in the molecular department which is my favorite. I've worked second shift in that department ever since. My particular area is molecular oncology and infectious disease using real time PCR and next generation sequencing (NGS). Because I participated in this program, I had no student debt.

What is the biggest challenge for you in your job? Is the shift a challenge?

The learning curve is steep in the beginning. I think troubleshooting is the most challenging aspect until you get thoroughly familiar with the instruments and sample problems. It's smoother now.

Is your job different since Covid? How did it affect you?

Covid was drastic. I put in tons of overtime. Once I worked five 12-hour shifts in a week and often worked four 12s. Sometimes, there was no time for meals and it was even difficult to take bathroom breaks. It was particularly difficult before I came to molecular because, early in the course of the epidemic while I was still

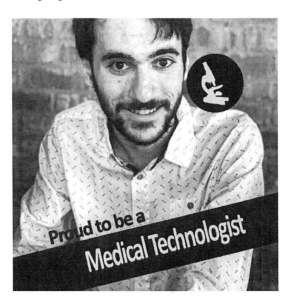

Eric Linney, MT

57

at the hospital, we had to call all positives and as many as 50 percent were positive. At that time, our results did not transfer to the computer so we had to hand enter them. That hospital lab could not use the batch testing we had in molecular so it was somewhat faster when I came to work in this department but it was still challenging and the testing volume was much higher.

Do you feel stressed in your job?

I don't find myself under as much stress now. There is just the pressure of knowing that what I do affects people's lives. Because I did phlebotomy, I remember many of those patients and it makes me more aware that there is a human being behind that sample.

If you feel stressed, is support of any kind offered in your place of work?

I get support from the other techs. I rely on my co-workers and they have been wonderful. I can honestly say that I have the support of my colleagues when needed.

How does it affect your home life?

I am getting married this year. My future spouse works at home so that makes it convenient because I still see her even though we work opposite shifts. I worked first shift for a little while when I was working as an LMA but I like second shift because of the shift diff. I work four ten hour shifts here in molecular. My fiancée and I want to have children and we plan to continue our working hours as they are so that one of us can always be at home for the kids.

Do you feel recognized as part of the healthcare team?

No one outside the medical field knows what I do and, when I try to explain it, I see their eyes glazing over. I finally just say that I am a scientist and I work in a medical facility. A career as a medical laboratory scientist is behind the scenes. Few people know we exist and many people assume doctors and nurses do the lab testing . They do not.

Do you feel satisfaction in you work?

Yes, I love my job. I had originally planned to get a PhD in genetics but I was getting burned out with continual school. This field is not without its stresses but I really enjoy my work in molecular. The oncology part involves using tumor samples from colon, lung or melanoma and doing genetic sequencing. Then, we work with a pathologist to ascertain the diagnosis, the prognosis and a therapy regimen targeted to that particular cancer rather than the one size fits all approach medicine used to have to use before this information was available, I want to keep learning and I hope to move up as I get more experience.

Would you recommend that young people go into this field? Why or why not? What would you tell them about the field?

If they like science and healthcare, I would tell them it is meaningful work. I have recommended the field to people who I think might do well in it. Most of the people I've talked to don't even know that the field exists. The online job description given on the hospital website makes it sound really dull. I tell them to pursue an internship or to at least talk to people who are actually doing the work before they decide about going into the field because it is not dull. It is anything but.

Six

A Lab of My Own

After I got my degree, I stayed on at both hospitals for a time but I had received my letter from AHCA (Agency for Healthcare Administration) certifying that I was now qualified to be a Medicare approved supervisor. I suppose I was a little intimidated, at first, because the job I took was not as a supervisor but rather as a lead tech. Lead techs take care of all the QC (quality control) and inhouse problems but, though they are usually included in interviewing prospective staff, they do not have to deal with staffing or attend meetings. This was a brand new hospital. Since it was not yet open, I got in on the writing of procedure manuals, the setting up of instruments and stocking.

Many reagents have to be refrigerated and there has to be a system of rotating, to make sure older reagents are used first and that a new reagent is not used before it is calibrated. Our analyzers were now able to run the different levels of calibrators and to draw the curve themselves but we had more tests to calibrate. Immediately after calibrating, controls had to be run to make sure all was well. It was my job to make sure notations were always made for any control value out of range and to watch for any "shift or trend" on the control charts. Laboratory science is a process of check and recheck, all for the benefit of the patient.

It was exciting to be in on the ground floor of a new hospital and the other techs and I set the lab up as we thought best. We were not doing microbiology since that went to our larger sister hospital in a neighboring town. My biggest challenge as lead was to insist that all techs be trained in all departments and be forced to rotate through them all on a regular basis. We were too small to allow any tech to work only in one specialty. There were complaints as one tech had only worked chemistry for years and did not want to branch out. He was finally convinced of the need, however, and I trained him to use our new Sysmex cell counter after I had gone to Chicago to be trained on it myself. Cell counters now gave us red cell count, white cell count, platelet count and hemoglobin. The hematocrit, the percentage of the blood that is cells, was calculated using the diameter and number of the red cells. We were still making and staining slides by hand. Our chemistry analyzer was made by Hitachi and could run batteries of tests on one sample. In a hospital lab, chem profiles are frequently interrupted in order to run stats. Stats are always run first and usually come with a label clearly designating them as stat. It doesn't take you long to recognize stat as a four letter word. I often suspected that some stats were not emergencies but rather a way for the doctor to get his results before he set off for his golf game.

We had a few phlebotomists in this hospital who drew blood and also spun the blood down in a centrifuge as necessary in order to get serum for chemistry tests. However, in the morning, the phlebs were busy collecting on the floors and we had to go out to draw if there was a stat. One morning, a lady came into the ER and stat bloodwork was ordered. I went to the ER and had no problem drawing her but, when I looked around to find the sharps container for my dirty needle, there was none to be found. The one I did see was overflowing and I realized that I would have to recap the needle, a process we were discouraged from performing because it is one more opportunity to put yourself in harm's way. Sure enough, I laid the needle cap down on the mattress beside the patient and prepared to slide the needle into it. Just at that time, the patient decided to turn over. She jostled the bed and the needle went into my finger. This was serious because AIDS was in full swing in 1991 and hepatitis was also a worry. I had to go through the protocol of being tested for both and retested at a specified time later. I was lucky as this lady only had pneumonia and I had no ill effects but it was a reminder that what we do is dangerous.

Another object lesson came when my fellow tech signed out the wrong blood. Mistakes are infrequent in laboratories because we have so many failsafes in place but they do occur. Because it is so important that blood transfusions be given only after the blood of the donor and of the recipient have been found to be compatible, we must be very careful to make sure that the unit which has been tested and assigned to that patient is the one which is actually given. The standard procedure is for the nurse to read off the patient's ID number and the patient group and type while the tech reads off the patient number and the specific number given to the unit of donor blood along with its group and type.

I don't know how the error occurred. Perhaps the numbers were very similar or the tech and/or nurse was overtired but the wrong unit went out. The patient had a transfusion reaction which can vary from itching with hives, fever and chills to more serious reactions involving blood in the urine, falling blood pressure or worse. This patient survived but it was a scary time for all of us. An incident report was generated, as required by law when there is an issue and the tech was written up and counseled.

Much money had been spent building and staffing this new hospital and money was running short. There were delays in deliveries but the worst part of the money shortage occurred on a weekend when I had a stat test ordered that we did not do inhouse. Our sister hospital ran that test and I called a cab to take the sample to that location. The cab did not come. When I called back, I was told that we had not paid the bill for the previous cab use. This was serious as this patient really needed this result. I called our pathologist and he came and got the sample himself but this kind of problem was worrisome. What if I couldn't reach the pathologist next time? This, along with the fact that we were sharing a supervisor with our sister hospital and I saw her once in the entire time I worked there, made me question whether I should continue in that hospital. I decided I should stop being afraid. If I was going to be supervising, I should take a position which would pay me for the work.

A supervisory job came up soon after in a group clinic. There were some GPs and oncology and hematology doctors in the practice. Along with supervising the lab, since it was small, I would be required to keep some accounts and print the payroll checks but I was prepared for that as I had kept the books for my husband's business during my marriage. I thought it would be a good place to try out my supervisory wings.

I learned far more about the business side of medicine than I did the clinical on this job. Until then, I had been blissfully ignorant of how bills got paid or even what was charged for any procedure. We had a woman who handled the billing but she was inexperienced and I found that I really needed to learn such matters myself.

What I learned is that there are three tiers to billing in the healthcare system. There is the amount the private insurance company will pay for any procedure, the amount Medicare will pay, and then the amount the patient will be expected to pay if he has neither. That amount is certain to be several times the amount either Medicare or private insurance will pay.

One website, https://khealth.com/learn/healthcare/how-much-does-bloodwork-cost/, gives a handy and up to date chart as to the relative costs of individual tests. For example, the hospital may charge $51 for a CBC. The insurance company will pay $11. Medicare will also pay $11. For a metabolic panel, which most of us get at least once yearly, the hospital charge may be $179, the insurance will pay $15 and Medicare $15. For a lipid profile, the charges are respectfully, $68, $29.99 and $29 (Vincenzo, 2022). I could go on but you get the point. The insurance companies have negotiated with individual labs to get the best price they can and that is why you are expected to use the lab your carrier demands. If you don't use that lab, your charges will be considerably more.

I have often heard people (usually people not in medicine) complain that people who use the ER don't pay their bills. Of course, the ER is grossly overused because people who don't have insurance can go there and the ER cannot refuse to treat them. But the truth is, even if the people want to pay their bills, the bills are so high that they can't pay them. That is because they are being charged the inflated rates which apply to patients who have neither insurance nor Medicare. And they pay these rates not just for lab tests but also for any other treatment. I know the info on this website is accurate because I am on Medicare and I see on my statements the greatly discounted rates my insurance company has arranged and the staggering difference between that amount and the amount the lab—or therapy or surgery—actually billed.

When I first became aware of this, I was stunned. My first thought was, if the lab can do the work of a CBC for $11, why are they charging $51, to someone off the street? Of course, some people will pay the $51 and never know that they're getting a bad deal. Also, the lab can write off that $40 they don't get (the difference between what they charged for a CBC and what they got) as loss. Of course, this tier system also applies to drugs and almost every other procedure in a hospital. No doubt, if some patients pay the inflated charges, that income helps to finance the people who never pay. Some hospitals have notices posted advising the uninsured that they can ask for discounted rates. They certainly should.

This lab is where I first became involved with computer entry. Our drawing station was up front and the chemistry analyzers were further down the hall. This was before lab results could be fed directly from the machines to a central computer. Prior to the recent purchase of this lab, the techs had just used the old fashioned way of handwritten lab slips. However, we were doing far more testing now and it is easier for the doctor if all results are on a limited number of papers. One of the biggest headaches was entering all the results into the computer.

My techs were good and they were hard workers but they had very little experience with large analyzers or with computers. It was a learning experience for all of us. I also found that it puts you outside the box when you are a supervisor. Though of course I liked some people especially, no favoritism can be shown and the same rules must apply for all.

Because of the AIDS epidemic, OSHA (Occupational Health and Safety Administration) had come up with new regulations requiring the wearing of disposable gloves when drawing blood or handling it in the lab. We also had to use face masks if there was a danger of splatter, such as when opening tubes. Some people were resistant as it is more difficult to find a vein when you have lost much of your tactile sense but I explained that it was permissible to find the vein first, then put on the gloves and do the draw and everyone accepted it.

My daughter had been admitted to the occupational therapy program at a Florida university. I went up to visit and liked what I saw of the town. I have always been an outside person and there was lots of green space there along with great clubs like Audubon and a native plant society. It has been my experience over the years that many med techs, nurses and doctors are drawn to the type of hobby which calls for things to be identified. It isn't difficult to understand why. Birds have different plumages at different stages just as cells do and the ability to identify a plant using key points is very like using key indicators to identify bacteria on a plate. I began to look into supervisory positions in the area.

Luck was with me. A reference lab in the university town was looking for a lab supervisor. I went for an interview and found that I really clicked with the operations manager. I was offered the job. I put in my notice at the clinic as soon as I returned and prepared to move. I even bought a house and three acres of land with the idea that my daughter would live with me and commute to class.

That's when my luck ran out. My mother was diagnosed with lung cancer. I was the only sibling living close and I knew I could not leave her at that time. I had already given notice and the lab was interviewing to replace me but they kindly let me stay on under the circumstances. Of course, I had to give up the new job which was a big disappointment. I had already bought the house and after I found out that I couldn't move at that time, my daughter had to take in roommates.

One advantage (or disadvantage) of working in medicine is that you can get the truth of any diagnosis if you want it. My mother had adeno-carcinoma of the lung. I asked our pathologist to please tell me truth-fully what the prognosis was. He told me it would be ten months to two years with treatment. She got ten months.

About the time of my mother's death, the manager of the lab where I had previously committed called me. It seemed that the supervisor they had hired in my place did not work out and the job was again open. Oh, happy day! I again gave notice at the clinic and they were beyond understanding. There was another woman who wanted the position at the clinic badly so it worked out for all.

I admit that I spent the first few weeks at my new job in something of a fog. It was so different! This was a reference lab. We ran many tests inhouse but there were many more to be sent out to a sister lab a hun-dred miles away. Our lab had a fantastic computer system. All samples that came in from the doctors and clinics who used our lab had their data entered and a unique accession number generated for that patient. The accession number would be the same on each tube for that number, but, depending on what tests were ordered, separate barcodes for each instrument would print out for that accession. So there would be a tube for the hematology analyzer, one for the chemistry analyzer and some samples had to be split so as to use another barcode for drug analysis or other special chemistry tests on a different machine.

Micro specimens got their own barcodes. Because some tests went to the sister lab where they would be run that night, the samples had to be accessioned, bar coded and prepared for running either inhouse or for sending out by a certain time every evening. Couriers would arrive at the specified time and it all had to be processed, packed in coolers and ready to go. The coolers had thermometers and either ice packs or dry ice so the quality of the sample could be assured. Temps of the coolers were taken and logged. Our couriers covered a large area and there were breakdowns. I left work at 6 p.m. but I got many calls at home when samples did not arrive on time. In that case, we had to either arrange for someone else to pick up the samples if there was time or I had to call the facilities on his route and inform them that the results would be delayed since the courier to the main lab did not wait.

We ran two shifts. The day shift mostly did stats and the work sent in by local doctors during the day. We also drew patients up front. The evening shift had the bulk of the work. The operations manager, Alice, was one of the most brilliant people I have ever known. Alice could think outside the box and come up with a plan C while we were all dithering about whether to go with A or B. We had one tech who was going home to the Philippines for three weeks and Alice asked me to work the bench while she was away. It was the best way to actually learn how things were done and it allowed me to find problems in the processes.

As a supervisor, I really liked being able to make needed changes. Some tests had minor computer glitches. Fields needed to be added or canned messages made available to eliminate typing the same comment over and over. Hemolysis is a big problem in the lab. When we only want to measure what is in the serum we want to eliminate what is within red cells. Red cell contents can be released into the serum if the phlebotomist does not have an uninterrupted flow. In a difficult draw, red cells rupture and spill their unwanted constituents into the serum, resulting in what we call hemolysis. If the test is a chemistry panel that includes potassium or several other analytes the value will be falsely elevated if the specimen is hemolyzed. The techs were having to type in a disclaimer about hemolysis every time as we needed to let the doctor know that the specimen was contaminated. If it was badly hemolyzed, we rejected the sample altogether. With the help of IT, we were able to formulate some canned messages and make reporting easier.

Electrolyte analysis had come a long way since the old flame photometer. We now used ISE (ion selective electrodes) to measure sodium, potassium and chloride. This was a great improvement and allowed these analytes to be measured as part of a panel or individually. One of the most common stat requests is for electrolytes. They run the electrical system of the body including control of heart rhythm and brain function. Dehydration can be a factor in abnormal electrolytes as can an overdose of potassium supplement. There was the case of a lady who thought more was better of her K-lyte and wound up in the ER with heart palpitations and chest pain, all from a greatly elevated potassium. Of course, we had to run known substances as controls daily to make sure our electrodes were working properly.

The biggest difference in working in a reference lab was the sheer mass of work. Speed and volume were the order of the day. Couriers brought the majority of work after the doctors' offices had closed. We also drew in nursing homes. It was a race to get it out the door by the time the courier came to pick it up. We had a group of processors who were part of my staff. They put the barcodes on the tubes after data entry had typed in the patient information and generated the barcodes. Of course, this had to be carefully done as mix-ups could occur if the wrong label was put on a tube. Today the barcodes are generated and put on the tubes while the patient is still in the drawing chair, eliminating that danger.

Early on, I noticed that data entry was mobbed when the couriers arrived from the doctors' offices and draw centers while processing was standing around, waiting on barcodes. I learned that the data entry clerks were not bringing the barcodes into processing until they had entered 24 patients. I asked why this was the magic number and they just gave me the old saw, "that's the way we've always done it." I really came to hate that phrase as no improvements can ever be made if people are resistant to change. I suggested that we begin bringing the barcodes into processing after only 12 patients had been entered and it made a big difference.

Because we got samples from prisons and other places with high incidence of AIDS, people had to be very careful with their PPE (personal protective equipment). I had one tech who was very resistant to wearing gloves. She even resorted to cutting the fingertips off the gloves. I never understood her objection as she did not draw and the gloves did not interfere with using the machines. After reminding her several times, I finally said to her, "Cathy, if you don't care whether you get the virus, how about your boyfriend?" Does he know you put yourself and indirectly, him, in jeopardy by refusing to wear gloves? That finally seemed to get the point across.

When I substituted for our Filipina tech, I began on urines. You may be familiar with the sticks we use to measure different chemicals in urine. In a low volume place, the tech just dips the stick into the urine by hand and waits the required time before reading the color changes visually. As a reference lab, we did not have the luxury of time. We had a machine into which we fed the strips after dipping them into the urine and the machine read the color changes in the blocks, telling the doctor whether the urine contained too much sugar, bilirubin or urobilinogen, white cells, blood, protein, nitrites (which are given off by certain bacteria) and ketones, which are given off by unregulated diabetics or by people who fast or go on low carbohydrate diets. The strips also gave us specific gravity. We saw high specific gravities in summer when people, especially men, exercised in the sun and didn't drink enough to compensate for perspiration. Lastly, they gave the pH, a measure of acidity. Bacteria are less likely to grow in acidic urine and pH affects the types of crystals seen under the scope.

After we got the reading from the machine, an aliquot of urine was spun down in a centrifuge and examined under the scope. Urine sediment was always checked for white cells and red cells which indicate infection. Strips today measure leukocyte esterase which gives an indication that we will likely see white cells. Crystals in urine can be calcium oxalate, which look like little envelopes or dumbbells, triple phosphate with their resemblance to coffin lids, or uric acid which take different shapes but mostly look like parallelograms and are often colored. These are all common and may mean nothing but too many CaOx crystals may indicate that kidney stones are forming and too many uric acid crystals may indicate gout. There are other crystals which are cause for alarm like cysteine or cholesterol crystals which indicate disease. Since urine can tell the doctor so much about the how the body is functioning, we had a lot of urines in this lab and it kept me busy for eight full hours just examining them.

Processing is a very important department in any lab but particularly so in a reference lab where doctors will expect their results the next morning. We had five or six processors opening bags, taking out the samples and separating them from the paper requisitions that came with them. The requisitions went to data entry where the data was typed in and barcodes printed which then went back to processing to be put on the specimens. Several of the processors were black. I was appalled when I first moved to Florida in 1958 at the age of 13 to see that black people could not sit down and eat with whites even though they were paying the same price for their food. In one restaurant back then, a plasterer, fresh off the job and covered in plaster, was obliged to go outside and eat his meal in the blazing sun while the rest of us sat in air conditioning. That was so wrong. The way our society works, however, we sometimes don't have the opportunity to get to know other races very well.

I made a point of participating in processing so as to understand how it worked and found that I really enjoyed the company of these workers. They were good natured even when busy and we could chat all evening about what we were going to have for supper. Not that they weren't ambitious. Many were in college and I had one young man who was brilliant. He had a degree in music and could name all the classical music composers and was now going to university for a microbiology degree. They were dependable and always contributed generously when we had a carry-in luncheon with terrific home-made food. I never sensed any racial tension among our group though the OJ Simpson case was in the news. Vocal opinions were expressed but it never escalated.

We had a send out department in this lab to enter data and pack up any specs which needed to go to a special reference lab. There's a lab in Triangle Park in North Carolina and esoteric tests could be sent there. Our send out clerk was a very bright Vietnamese-American young man who would later go on to medical school. I've always thought it is desirable to keep both alive if you happen to belong to two cultures. He was thoroughly American but he participated in a Vietnamese club. We went to a fundraiser where we learned to eat Pho and he told us about their New Year's festivity where he was the ass half of the dragon. His could be a challenging job because the university in our community had a large medical school and the doctors there attended lectures and were privy to new medical discoveries. Sometimes they ordered tests which were not even in the catalog yet. There would be a rash of the same unusual test ordered and our joke was that "the doctors have read another article."

Any manager will tell you that staff management is the toughest part of the job and this job was no exception. It only takes one person "stirring the pot" to create havoc and we had a few. In the beginning I was in charge only of the lab and processing but over time it became reasonable for me to take on data entry because they worked so closely with processing. This meant I had to follow how many accessions each person was entering. Our computer system made this possible because we all had unique passwords. One person either could not or did not meet the requirement despite verbal and written warning. He was belligerent when I had to let him go and I was grateful that the courier supervisor sat in on the meeting as it was the first firing for me. We also had one person who was gunning for another person's job and it was a source of constant conflict. They both wound up leaving.

Because it was a university town, we had what I began to call the semester shuffle. When the semester began, all the people who wanted to take day courses now wanted to work evenings and those that had night classes wanted day shift. I struggled to accommodate everybody but it could be a hassle. Being students, they were all part-time and it made for a larger number of employees than if they had all been fulltime workers. At one time, I had the responsibility of fifty people.

In the lab, I was blessed with mature experienced techs and I found after some time on the job that they were not making salaries commensurate with techs elsewhere. I obtained data from other labs and was able to get raises for them that were richly deserved.

Our computer system was called Antrim and it was a marvel. We even had normal values for canines and felines. We received samples from vets and sometimes from the vet school. There was an entry blank in Antrim for species. Data entry would specify that it was a cat or a dog rather than a human and the report would print out with the correct normal range for that species. This all worked beautifully until our marketing rep engineered a contract with an ostrich farm. Of course, she did not know that the red cells of birds and reptiles, unlike those of humans, still have a nucleus. Our instruments counted all the red cells as lymphocytes. We could not get usable results on these birds and our volume was far too great to be doing manual counts so we had to let that contract go. She also arranged for us to do blood counts on bat blood. The samples were tiny micro tubes and were often clotted. The techs complained, with reason. Late in the year she took several of us out for a meal at the Melting Pot. I felt that we had earned it.

While I was in Indianapolis training on a new chemistry analyzer, I got a call from Alice. She began by saying, "you don't work for the same company you worked for when you left." Our lab had been taken over by a larger multi-state reference lab. This transition was no doubt the most challenging period of my entire career. The new lab's computer system at that time did not even use barcodes. We had to print large sheets of numbers of many digits and affix each individually to the tubes. Instead of each specimen being barcoded when it went on the instrument, techs had to print worksheets and line the specimens up in the exact order of the worksheet, then accept all the results as a batch.

It was truly a large step backwards. If a specimen happened to be reversed, wrong results could be transmitted. Added to that, the new parent lab did not use the same instruments and there was no computer program written to link our instruments to the computer. We had been told that this would be done before we went "live," meaning the actual reporting of patient results. That day arrived and nothing worked. I had paid to attend my high school reunion that day but it was not to be. One tech, dependable Beth, and I worked the entire weekend hand entering hundreds of results. I shall be eternally grateful for her help.

Then began the search for lost specimens and, without the assurance of barcodes, there were far too many, Every day I would print a list of pending results and start attempting to track them down. I would spend a great deal of time on the phone with the person at the parent lab while she searched on her end for missing numbers. We were all disappointed in the system as we had found comfort in the idea of specimen integrity when each barcode was specific. Now we all had to check and recheck that the numbers on the worksheet corresponded exactly with the lineup of tubes on the machine before any batch could be released. If the machine missed reading a sample for some reason, that number had to be identified and deleted from the worklist before results could go out. I had irate calls from doctors because results were delayed or simply missing and I got very good at groveling. All I could do was explain the situation and assure them that we were working out the bugs.

In time, we adjusted to the new system as it did no good to sit around grieving for Antrim. After things settled down, I was able to attain one last goal of my professional life. I sat for and passed the medical technology exam for ASCP (the American Society of Clinical Pathologists), in 1994. This is a national registry and is the most prestigious of registries as it is recognized all over the country. This allowed me to put the coveted letters after my name, MT, ASCP. Alice ordered an ASCP pin for me, something I treasure to this day.

Instrumentation had been greatly improved over time and one technology for which we were particularly grateful was the methodology for measuring protimes (prothrombin times). If we had been obliged to rock tubes looking for clotting as we did in the old days, we most certainly would never have gotten the work out. Instead, the new method involved a machine that had probes which could sense when a clot was forming, not only speeding up the process but also removing the factor of human vision differences. Protimes are very important as patients in danger of throwing a clot were usually put on Coumadin, the main component of which is warfarin. Warfarin was discovered by a veterinarian in 1939 when he noticed that cattle who fed on sweet clover often hemorrhaged. The clover was analyzed and warfarin was isolated. It works by blocking some of the clotting factors we have already mentioned (Lim, 2014).

The object behind anticoagulant theory is to thin the blood enough to avoid clots without thinning it too much. The protime also tells the doctor if the dosage is adequate as it should not be normal during anti-coagulant therapy. During my time at the reference lab, the INR came into use. Previously, we had reported protimes out only in seconds. This method was not used all over the world so we began using the International Sensitivity Index which made it possible for all methods and all reagents to be comparable (Horsti, 2009). Newer methods of anti-coagulation have been invented but coumadin is still in use and it is vitally important that patients on this drug be tested regularly. My own mother-in-law died from excess coumadin that had built up in her system. She died of blood loss before it could be arrested. She had not been going for her blood tests sufficiently often.

In every lab, we begin the day with taking temperatures. Every fridge must come within a certain limit as well as every freezer. All temps are logged and the logs must be available during inspections. This is especially critical in blood bank. Twice during my career, I did find that fridges were not working properly and valuable reagents might have been lost if we had not done due diligence. There is a great deal of record keeping in the clinical lab. Control values were now transmitted directly from the instrument into the computer system so there was no "fudging" control values. The computer system would flag if the control was not within range. Action logs were scrutinized to make sure tech action was documented for any control value out of range. Control graphs are printed every month routinely but I, as supervisor, didn't wait until the end of the month to find out if our values were within range. Means had to be recalculated periodically and charts adjusted due to new lots of reagents or other changes.

Day shift received a lot of stats as we had contracts with certain doctors who expected to get quick results when time was of the essence. Protimes, CBCs, urinalysis and blood glucose were common stats but we also did drug levels. Probably the most common drug to be tested was digitalis, a drug given to improve heart function. Overdose can cause palpitations among other more serious effects and not taking enough defeats therapy. We also ran phenytoin, better known as Dilantin and phenobarbital, both given to control seizures. Patients do not always take drugs as directed and the doctors need to know if the blood level is within therapeutic range.

We got liver panels consisting of LDH (lac dehydrogenase), SGOT, now known as AST (aspartate aminotransaminase), and SGPT, now known as ALT (alanine aminotransferase), GGT (glutamyl transpeptidase), ALP (alkaline phosphatase), total protein, albumin and bilirubin. Before I trained, I really didn't know what our livers do for us. The liver is considered to be a gland, which was news to me. The liver produces bile which is stored in the gallbladder. Bile aids in the digestion of fats and fat soluble vitamins. Vitamin K cannot be absorbed without the assistance of the liver so it is important for the clotting of blood. The greenish brown color of bile is caused by bilirubin and biliverdin, products of the breakdown of old red blood cells.

The liver eliminates these and other toxic substances from the body (Hole, 1978). Think alcohol metabolism. Earlier, I mentioned jaundice in liver cancer. Another reason for jaundice is if the bile duct is blocked, such as happens in gall bladder disease, the bile backs up and turns the skin yellow. Because the liver is important in the clotting of blood, a protime was sometimes included in a liver profile. Any of the tests ending in ase are enzymes and some enzymes can be elevated in liver disease, whether it was from hepatitis or cirrhosis or secondary to a blocked bile duct.

Two more enzymes we ran were amylase and lipase which are elevated in pancreatitis. Doctors depend on these lab results to decide whether the patient has pancreatic malfunction and they are often ordered stat because the patient is in so much discomfort.

We ran a lot of lipid profiles, consisting of total cholesterol, HDL, triglycerides and a calculated LDL—which can be run as a direct measurement but is usually just a calculation. The formula is total cholesterol–HDL–triglycerides divided by five. I will give my latest lab result to clarify. My total cholesterol was 180. My HDL was 60. My triglycerides were 90, calculation LDL=181–60–90/5=103.

Kidney function is usually measured via BUN (blood urea nitrogen) and creatinine. The BUN can vary somewhat but both it and creatinine, which is derived as waste from muscle action, should be cleared by the kidneys. If kidney function is inadequate, BUN and creatinine build up in the blood. Albumin, one form of protein in the blood, should not ordinarily be excreted and albumin in the urine is another indicator that the kidneys are not working at full capacity. They are supposed to retain protein and the right amounts of electrolytes and eliminate the rest. If the tiny tubules of the kidneys are damaged, such as in uncontrolled high blood pressure, proteins that the body still needs are not retained and toxic substances that should be excreted build up in the blood.

Our second shift ran all of the above tests but lots more of them. Having the tests run inhouse got the results to the doctor faster but it required at least three techs to man it. The newly merged lab was a business and it was decided at some point that our second shift would be eliminated and their work sent to the parent lab. I still had my duties of quality control, making sure we had procedures written for every test and presiding over staff and inspections but it was not the same without the second shift and I was ready to move on.

Interview with a New Supervisor (2023)

Name, shift and duties, how long have you worked in the lab?

My name is Nancy Tartaglia. I work at a hospital and am the new lab manager, working days. I began my lab career as a laboratory medical technician in 1984. After I moved to Florida, I took further classes. Those classes plus my years of experience allowed me to sit for the technologist exam.

What is the biggest challenge for you in your job? Are the hours or shifts a challenge?

Being a supervisor is new to me. I am expected to attend meetings and deal with inspections. I was already familiar with inventory and ordering as well as technical issues as a bench tech but staffing concerns are up to me now. We have a great group now at my lab but we are still using traveling techs until I can find more qualified techs.

Is your job different since Covid? How did it affect you during the epidemic?

Covid went on for a very long three years. It was so stressful. Our techs did a great job. Everyone pitched in and we depended on each other. The break room was the place to commiserate. We could curse or laugh together because we were all under pressure to get the tests out. I just kept thinking, one patient at a time. Keep it up and get it done!

Do you feel stressed in your job? If so, do you have some on-the-job support?

People tend to be resistant to change but I ask for suggestions from longtime staff. I find that staff will accept change if they see that the process improves. We have had to use traveling techs for more than a year. Because they come from a company that provides emergency staffing, the company gets a cut and it is expensive. We are looking for new hires. It seems that the new generation of workers wants fulfillment where I just wanted stability. Of course, everyone wants to be treated well but their expectations seem to be higher than mine were at that stage of my career. I always have someone I can call if I have questions. Hospital administration has been supportive.

How does your work affect home life? Do you find it difficult to balance work and the rest of life? How do you handle childcare, if applicable?

I first worked in a private lab on night shift because I did not have to work weekends or holidays there. I had three kids so that was important to me and, by working night shift, my husband and I could care for the kids. It wasn't easy. I would come home in the early morning, sleep for an hour, then wake up and get the kids to school, then sleep another few hours before I had to go back to work. Later, I went to work in another lab on second shift. After I moved to Florida, I went to work in the hospital weekend shifts: Friday, Saturday and Sunday. I kept this kind of shift for 15 years. My children are now grown and it gives me satisfaction that my husband and I did it together.

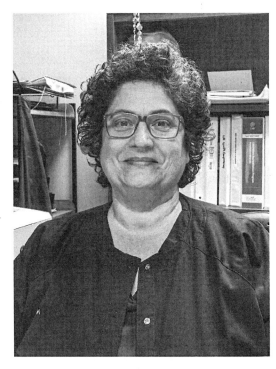

Do you feel that you are recognized as part of the healthcare team?

I did feel that our work was not recognized by the outside world during Covid. But internally, it's better in the last five years. The pay has become more commensurate. In this job,

Nancy Tartaglia, MT

75

as a manager, I have to learn to give and take. Though my hospital is not for profit, it still has to be run as a business. We have to be concerned with production and I have to keep track of how well we are doing individually and as a department in the healthcare system.

Do you feel satisfaction in your work? Are you glad you went into the field?

Yes, absolutely. I can't imagine doing anything else. This job has supported my family all these years. My husband works in construction. He didn't always have access to medical insurance but I could count on it in my job. If he was without work, I still had my paycheck.

Would you recommend young people go into this field? Why or why not? What would you tell them about the field?

Yes, it's a great profession. My sisters work in healthcare but I found that I didn't really like patient contact. Now, probably 99 percent of the new trainees don't even learn to draw blood so, if they would rather work behind the scenes like me, this is a good job for them. Also, there are other places to work once you become an experienced tech. I know people who have become reps for the instrument companies, or they work in the call centers helping techs over the phone when they have instrument issues. And you can always get a job. There are openings all over in the lab.

SEVEN

The Hospital Lab:
Where the Action Is

After I decided to leave the reference lab, I put my house up for sale in 1997. It did not sell right away and I was looking for something to do in the interim. I took a job at a small hospital about 45 minutes away which was experiencing staffing problems. After I took the job of supervisor, I realized that the person serving as lab director knew he needed to "clean house" but was unwilling to do it. He had one tech who really could not be trusted to do the work. She was rude to other staff, she drank to excess and she had to go. Another one, who was a good friend to the first, left soon after.

That took care of one problem but I also found that the procedure manuals on the shelves were not even the right manuals for the instruments they were using. Lots of typing followed and I often had to work the bench in lieu of the missing techs. This hospital was the one place where I was obliged to take call during my career. We had no third shift so we rotated through call for any stat orders that came in at night. At first, I would go home after a call out but soon found that, while I was enroute, I would too often have received a call to come in again. This was before the age of cell phones.

One memorable night, I was called to do a CBC on a young man who was having a serious bleed. To my disbelief, his hemoglobin was slightly over five grams. The red cells themselves were normal but he simply had less than half the normal amount of blood due to alcoholism and bleeding. We did not have an in-house blood bank but we did have blood on the shelves and a system whereby we sent a sample of blood from the patient to a sister lab. The sister lab had retained a little section of the tubing from each of the units of blood in our fridge called a pigtail. The segment contained the same blood as that in the bag. They then crossmatched the sample we sent with the "pigtail" which they had retained. The sample from our patient had to be couriered to the sister hospital. I had to wait for the results before the blood could be issued and, needless to say, I was there most of the night.

Every hospital laboratory that accepts Medicare must be certified by some agency accepted by CLIA, adhering to CLIA standards. This inspection was done by the Joint Commission on Accreditation of Healthcare Organizations. I got them through the JCAHO inspection that they had been dreading and received flowers for my efforts but I knew I couldn't handle that place any longer.

My father was still living further south in Florida. He was remarrying and his place was up for sale. I decided to buy it, which was good for him and it gave me a place to live while I was looking for my next job. Though I would later regret it, I decided against trying for a supervisory position. I suppose I was burnt out at the time. Instead, I took a PRN (as needed) job at a hospital in a nearby town. I loved it from the start. The techs were very helpful, and they were glad to have someone they could call on if they were sick or just needed time off. Many of the instruments were familiar and the instruments were connected to a laboratory computer system which then connected to the hospital computer system, eliminating most hand entry of results. Each instrument had its own computer and each one had a different way of interacting with it. Some required a mouse, some had a track ball, some had a touch pad and some used a touch screen. I often felt it was like knowing multiple languages. Our brains just kicked in with the right muscle memory as soon as we began to work on that machine.

I had taken COBRA from my last job. That is extended health insurance from my previous employer for which I had to pay the employer portion as well as my own. COBRA can only be taken for 18 months and my time was running out. I knew I would have to take fulltime employment soon to get health insurance. I really wanted to work in microbiology. There was a hospital close to my home and they did have a micro department so I applied to work in that department. I waited and waited until one day the supervisor of chemistry at this hospital called me and said that she had just recently seen my application and noted that I was licensed in all departments. There was no opening in micro but she wanted to know if I would be willing to work in chemistry. I took the job and thus began what I feel was the happiest period in my career.

Both the hospital where I had worked as a PRN and the one where

I took a fulltime job were not-for-profit hospitals. By this time, I had worked in both for-profit and not-for-profit hospitals. I have heard some people say that they would rather go to a for-profit hospital because the for-profits are not obliged to take the indigent. As I understand it, any ER is obliged to take all who come unless they are just too full which does happen in the winter in Florida when even a 50-bed ER can be overloaded and patients must be taken to another ER. But they must be seen somewhere. In the case of the hospital group where I worked, they are taken to another hospital in the system if possible or to wherever the patient wants to go.

In order to retain their tax exempt status, not-for-profits must care for the indigent, and there is no doubt that they often absorb that cost without being recompensed. Since a large number of people in the U.S. have no medical insurance, this can be a drain on hospitals' resources. (Levinson, 2022). For-profit hospitals must see all ER patients and they do provide care for some indigents but the for-profit systems have shareholders who expect to make a profit on their investment. In my experience, the not-for-profits have been better staffed and better equipped than their for-profit counterparts. I believe that is because the profit going to shareholders might otherwise go into newer machinery or more staffing.

I began my new job on second shift which is usually 2:30 p.m. until 11 p.m. We rotated through five benches. Urinalysis alone was a teaching experience. Of course, I had examined body fluids and done semen analysis at other places but not in the quantity I now saw in this large hospital which also had outreach clients such as we had at the reference lab. One evening I ran 80 urines and did five body fluids. A body fluid may be a spinal fluid from a spinal tap or an aspirate from a knee or toe or elsewhere. In spinal fluid the doctor is looking for white cells such as those found in meningitis. Chemistries are run on the spinal fluid, too. Excess protein along with decreased sugar in the sample indicates bacterial infection while little or no change in either is likely to mean viral meningitis. In taps from joints, the doctor is looking for the cause of inflammation. We may find white cells indicating infection or we may find crystals such as those found in gout. To identify crystals properly we used a special polarizing filter which was attached to our microscope.

Different crystals rotate light in different directions. That fact plus the appearance of the crystal allows us to determine what kind of crystal it is. This is important because some conditions mimic gout and identifying the correct crystal verifies the diagnosis. It is a time-consuming process to fit the filter to the scope, then look over the whole field for crystals and, of course, all other work is waiting while this is being done. On the same evening I got a semen analysis.

We commonly looked at post-vasectomy specimens in which you do not expect to find any sperm and they are easy but a full-fledged semen analysis is not. It was not usual for these to come in on second shift when we had so much work to do but there it was and a semen analysis cannot wait. After noting the viscosity and general appearance of the semen, you then look at the sample under the scope to determine motility of the spermatozoa and whether there are abnormal forms. Then you need to count the sperm to see if there is an adequate num-ber. To count them, you first have to make them stay still. We did this by putting an aliquot in the freezer for a time.

At the same time we set up motility studies. Small samples are sealed within coverslips and then left on a heating block set to body temp. They have to be examined at specified intervals to make sure the sperm maintain motility over time. While they are heating, some other work gets done until the semen specimen in the freezer has had time to thoroughly chill. Then it is time to take the sample out of the freezer and count the sperm. This is done under the microscope on a ruled count-ing chamber such as we used in the past for white cells or on a Mak-ler chamber specific for the purpose. The specimen is diluted to make it easier to count.

You can't delay in the counting process as the sperm cells are warming up all the time. After the count is done, there is a formula to use to account for the dilution and the size of the chamber. Though this may be taking a lot of your time, the same care must be taken as if you had all the time in the world as some couple who wants a child is wait-ing on the result.

One thing I liked about this lab were the windows. They opened only to a second wall but some kind person had planted crepe myrtles between the buildings so there was light and green outside to relieve the sterile atmosphere of the lab. We could see the changing of the seasons in their branches, a reminder that life went on, even when we were sur-rounded by sickness and death. At one time, we had a lab fish. Day shift techs made up a maintenance schedule for the fish just as we had for the instruments. It was nice to have a beautiful living thing in the lab but maybe the maintenance schedule wasn't adhered to or the fish had some other problem. For some reason, the fish died.

This hematology laboratory had an automatic slide stainer so we did not have to individually stain our slides for doing differentials. The hematology instrument had auto feed, meaning we put the tubes on and they went into the machine, the proper amount of blood was aspirated and the results printed out next to the computer station. The tech in charge of that department released the results or held them if there was a critical value or there was some reason to believe that the sample was not usable. It might be because of a clot or hemolysis. These labor saving machines are wonderful but they have their problems. Clots could form in the anticoagulated tubes during draws and the machine had to be bleached and rinsed to rid it of the obstruction. The belt on the slide stainer could jam and break slides. We were expected to call the hotline for any instrument not working and follow through with any suggestion the hotline made.

Every effort was made not to call for service. We had service contracts so it wasn't the money. It was the delay in results that was worrisome. Every machine had a backup method but they were usually smaller and slower. Controls were run on backup methods every shift so they would be ready to go if needed. We were so busy on second shift that one tech sat at the scope and did nothing but manual differentials all night. Another tech put the purple top tubes used for hematology on the instrument, examined the results and issued the report and did the same for coag with the blue top tubes. We had predetermined critical values and, if a critical value was found on review, it had to be called to the floor or, if it was an outpatient, to the ordering doctor. This was necessary but it used up time. The eternal paradox of lab work is that it must be accurate, but they want it yesterday.

I loved the people I worked with on second shift and we had a great supervisor. Nora's door was always open and you got the feeling that she actually cared about what you had to say. Her dedication was evident when she came into hematology one evening. She was heavily pregnant with her first child and I knew, from experience, that she had to be tired by that time of night. Fred and I were going on about some minor problem and she listened, but suddenly interrupted. "I don't want to be rude," she said, "but I think my water just broke." Indeed, it had and she went directly to labor and delivery with Fred in tow, all minor lab issues instantly forgotten.

Chemistry used large analyzers made by Beckman at the time. Chem profiles rolled off the analyzer by the hundreds. Every report had to be perused for either abnormal results or for any sign of a bubble, hemolysis or other problem that might cause an erroneous result. People with very high values had to have their sample diluted until we could obtain a valid result because, as in the old days, assays had curves. The underlying methodology was the same. The computer was drawing the curves after we ran the calibration solutions but they still had limits. If the sample was too high to be read on that curve it had to be diluted until it came within readable range. One problem was with patients who had very high lipids (fats) in their blood. I have seen blood serums with such high triglycerides that, instead of a normal yellow clear fluid, the serum looked like milk. These specimens had to be diluted and a message sent to the doctor that the specimen was highly lipemic. We did have a special high-speed centrifuge that could eliminate much of the lipemia if necessary.

In the case of enzymes, the methodology is to use a substrate that the specific enzyme breaks down. An example would be using starch to measure the activity of amylase. In disease states, there could be so much enzyme in the sample that the substrate being used to measure the reaction was used up immediately and the sample had to be diluted until it was not too much for the substrate. Sometimes, this took several sequential dilutions since, if that patient had not been run before, you had no way of knowing whether the sample would read diluted by two or if it was going to have to be diluted by 100. In these early days, we usually had what we called "report" at the end of the evening when there was an overlap between shifts so that we could tell the next tech about such patients. As costs went up and Medicare reimbursement went down, overlaps were eliminated and I often left the lab with sticky notes stuck all over the computer monitor, telling the next tech about Patient X and how much I had to dilute his sample.

Troponins had come into use by now and they were a big improvement for detecting heart attacks, especially in patients who did not come in right away. The CK was the wonder test when I trained and it is still measured but as a specific part of the enzyme, CK-MB (creatine kinase–myocardial band). Within 24 hours CK peaks in the blood and is gone within two to three days. CK and troponin are both enzymes released into the blood when there is damage to the heart muscle.

However, troponin is more specific, as CK is found in other muscles and other conditions can also lead to a high CK.

The patient you met earlier who had his beehive fall off the truck had a high total CK because of damage to the skeletal muscle from having a heavy beehive land on him. Troponin is specific to the heart so we say it has better specificity and sensitivity, two words we used often when evaluating new tests. Troponin can still be detected days after a heart attack and, since our town had a high number of people over the age of 65 and since heart disease is still the number one killer of people in the U.S., we ran a lot of troponins.

I once had an elevated troponin result pop up on my screen that belonged to a dear friend who had been a classmate in junior high, so a friend of long duration. We are not allowed, per HIPAA law (CDC, HIPAA, 2022), to give out any patient information we see in the lab. I called my friend later and she told me about the heart attack but I could not tell her that I had known in advance. We had to be very careful about discussing cases when in the dining room or in the elevator. Names could not be mentioned. Blabbing patient information could be grounds for dismissal. We also had to be very careful when faxing patient info to the doctor or nursing home. A wrong number could lead to a lawsuit.

Special chemistry was a fifth department at the time. Troponins and many other tests were done via immunoassay. This method is based on the antigen/antibody reaction talked about before. Berson and Yalow first described the method in 1959 and it earned them the Nobel prize in 1984. If the antigen is the substance to be detected, corresponding antibodies are used to find it. Often, these antibodies are developed by injecting the antigen into mice, which then develop the antibodies (Wu, 2006). If you are looking for the antibody, as when you want to know if a patient has already had chicken pox, you use the corresponding antigen (in this case, an extract from the chicken pox virus). The antigen or antibody which is added is tagged with a fluorescent molecule. If, indeed, the substance being searched for binds with the antigen or antibody added, the fluorescent tag is activated. The machine, which is closed like a black box so no light can come in from the outside, will detect the fluorescence and thus the presence of the desired substance is ascertained. In the case of enzymes such as troponin, the amount of fluorescence can be calculated to give a numerical level.

Some pregnancy tests were also done via immunoassay. We still had the little kit tests that were done on urine as a screening but, when the doctor suspected pregnancy, we ran quantitative HCG (human chorionic gonadotropin) on the machine and were able to give the doctor a numerical value which corresponded to the number of months pregnant. Tests for the antibodies to the hepatitis virus were run on this machine as well as testing for the antibodies to contagious diseases such as German measles. This test is always done on pregnant women as German measles during early pregnancy can cause birth defects.

Drug levels are often done via immunoassay. As new drugs came on the market, manufacturers of tests had to keep up. Gabapentin came out in 1993. It was originally used for seizure control. Now it is also used for relieving the pain of shingles and other conditions. Of course, we needed to start testing for that drug so the doctor could know if the patient was compliant and how it was being metabolized in that patient's body. We also tested for several antibiotics because some are toxic in high doses and not everyone clears the antibiotic from their system in a timely manner, particularly older people.

Then there were the recreational drug screens. Our hospital was the closest hospital to the beach. Friday and Saturday nights could be expected to bring several drug tests. It wasn't uncommon to learn that a car had come careening into the ER entrance and the patient pushed out into the parking lot, before the car tore off, so the driver couldn't be asked any questions. This left the doctor knowing that the patient was drugged but with no idea which drug. Drug screens were always stat and you dropped whatever you were doing to run them. At the time, we tested for amphetamines, opiates, marijuana, phenobarbital, benzodiazepines and cocaine.

The tests were done on urine via cards impregnated with an antibody to each drug. A positive showed up in a little window on the card next to the drug that was positive. It was something of a game to see how many positives would be detected on one card. I remember getting a quinella (five) on one patient. Since some of the drugs are sedatives, some hallucinogens, and some energizers, that patient couldn't have known whether he was up or down. I never knew anyone to get six positives on one patient but I'm sure it must have happened. As new recreational drugs came into being, manufacturers scrambled to get test kits out. For a time, we could not test for Ecstasy but you can now, along with ketamine, PCP, methamphetamine and others.

Then, there were the blood alcohols. Our lab had stopped drawing alcohol levels for law enforcement purposes. I understood why they had decided against getting involved in legal alcohols because I had drawn one at the small lab I worked at in North Florida and wound up having to drive two hours one way, months later, in order to testify in court that yes, that was my handwriting on the tube, and yes, the defendant was the person I drew the blood from. We did draw and run them for diagnostic purposes. In Florida the legal limit is 0.08 BAC (blood alcohol concentration). I have run levels as high as 0.4, five times over the limit. Alcohols were usually run along with drug screens as the two seem to go together.

Occasionally, we would have carry-in dinners. We arranged it so that day shift would still be around and second shift would come in a little early so that all could participate. I had enjoyed the ethnic food at other hospitals but this place was a real melting pot. I worked with a Korean woman who made wonderful glass noodles. Filipinas brought in those lovely fluffy dumplings with Bar-B-Q in the centers. We had Mexican-American, Norwegian, Vietnamese, Polish, Serbian-American, Indian, Colombian, Peruvian and Chinese-American techs, a tech from the Caribbean (I am still using her recipe for banana bread) and other techs from regions all over the States.

I remember one funny culture clash. Fred was a senior tech from Alabama and had been raised to always allow ladies to enter the door first. Giann was from Korea and had been raised to always allow the older person to go through the door first. This left them at an impasse one evening when they returned from dinner at the same time since each was waiting on the other. Finally, Fred said, "Giann, one of us is going to have to break tradition and go through the door or we're never going to get any work done." Though the work was serious, we had our laughs and laughter is the same in all languages.

We seldom saw doctors inside the lab on second shift. The pathologist would visit during day shift and the occasional hematologist would come in to look at a patient's slide but we generally worked on our own with only a senior tech or two for guidance. Second shift put out the majority of the work as the draws from the outreach clients came in after doctors' offices closed. We had to wait on processing to get the samples to us and, as it had been at the reference lab, that could be a holdup. One night a doctor came in asking why his patient's results had not been done. In fact, I didn't even have the sample. I explained to him that we couldn't run it if we didn't have it. He asked what was causing the delay. I didn't want to throw processing under the bus as I didn't know what problems they were encountering but I did assure him that the delay was not on the technical side. He could see that no one was sitting around and my supervisor reported to me the next day that the doctor was very impressed. I always tried to be professional as you can't expect people to treat you as a professional if you don't behave like one. I have worked in labs where bad language and yelling are commonplace. That kind of thing is not acceptable and it adds to the stress.

It was during this period that the hospital started offering some stress reduction options. One was the opportunity to get chair massages. When the masseuse started working on my shoulders, I realized how tight my muscles were. The massage helped but, more than that, it was validation that we did, indeed, feel stressed and that the hospital recognized it.

Another way we had to come together and enjoy camaraderie in a stress free environment was the invention of Lab Week. According to records, Lab Week actually began in 1975 but it was the 1990s before it spread around the country and was implemented at a hospital where I worked. It always took place in April and we all looked forward to that week every year. Supervisors never had a large budget to make it festive but senior techs and others would come up with fun things. There were contests and quizzes. The baby picture contest where we had to guess the tech's identity by looking at their baby picture was one of the best. One year I took pictures of the techs on my shift and we displayed them in the dining room. The idea was to make patients and staff aware that this small army of workers was down there and had faces.

Most of all, there was food. One of our pathologists was a part owner in a bagel company. During one day of Lab Week, as well as other times, he would provide bagels of all different kinds, along with spreads. Lab supply vendors would bring in pastries or even a whole lunch during Lab Week. We always had a carry-in luncheon that brought out the great variety of culinary dishes of all nationalities. The hospital would always provide some kind of Lab Week gift. I still have cups and water bottles with quotes honoring lab professionals as well as beach blankets, towels and pins. We had all experienced Nurses Week and it was gratifying to have a week of our own.

Sometimes we laughed our way through stress. We had a lab aide at the time. Her name was Ada and Ada washed all the myriad pipettes and other glassware that we used on all shifts. Ada was a lovely lady and I don't think we appreciated her sufficiently until she went on vacation.

We were spoiled by always having everything we needed close at hand and no one realized that we were running out of pipettes until halfway through second shift. Another tech, Linda, and I had to go into Ada's work room and figure out how to do this stuff that I had not done for many years and likely, Linda, who was much younger, had never done at all. There was a gizmo that you attached to the faucet which was supposed to send water through the pipettes, first with soap, then rinse water. We couldn't seem to get it sealed properly. It was a comedy of errors and we had water on the floor, the counters and on ourselves trying to get that hose hooked up to the faucet to do the washing. Of course, other techs were stuck with doing some of our work while we were playing Ada. It was funny at the time but I told Ada how much we had missed her when she returned.

Linda was an amazingly talented artist. Though she was a good tech, I often wonder if her creativity wasn't wasted in the lab. When I was a supervisor I did use some creativity in endeavoring to make things run more efficiently. But a bench tech must follow procedures as written. One tech told me that the right side of his brain, which is the creative side, had turned to mush. He said he couldn't brush his teeth without a procedure. It could be stultifying at times to have to follow the dots exactly.

Eventually, Ada retired and the hospital did not replace her. We went almost completely to disposable pipettes and threw them out after using. I understood the reasoning but the lab really does contribute a lot of waste. The waste had to be separated into red bag trash that is contaminated and ordinary paper which could go into regular trash. The red bags were in boxes, clearly marked and we had to close these up when full and another hospital team incinerated them. I have heard of red bag garbage being found in landfills but that never happened anywhere I worked.

During my tenure, our hospital merged with several hospitals to form a new consortium. It made sense since we could all use the same machines and the same reagents, making it possible to buy in bulk, saving money. It also made it possible for us to borrow from each other if we ran short. Some departments in the smaller hospitals were eliminated and the work sent to the larger hospitals as a streamlining measure. Of course, this meant tech positions were lost in the smaller hospital and, if the tech wanted to keep working for the new grouping, they were obliged to drive to the larger hospital that was getting the work. There were other adjustments. In the hematology and chemistry departments, it was decided that space was needed for Blood Bank so hematology and chemistry, which had been in two separate rooms, had to be combined. We called it chematology.

It was unavoidable but the one real downside was the noise. Any lab is noisy but having six large analyzers in the same room with their clicking and alarms along with the timers, phones and intercom could be nerve-wracking. Because the lab management really seemed to care about us, they installed sound proofing on as many surfaces as could be managed and it did help. What made it a good place to work, however, was not the concern of the management, though that was as it should be. It was the sense of teamwork. It was a busy place but we worked together. I dare not mention names lest I leave someone out but I remember them all fondly. I was never afraid to ask for help if I needed it and other techs would ask me for help in turn.

A hospital lab must be staffed seven days a week, 24 hours a day unless they are relying on techs coming in on call, a practice seldom seen today. We had a death of one of our night shift techs while I was at this hospital. Until a replacement could be hired, we had to split that shift between day shift and evening shift. I had to stay until 3 a.m. when it was my turn and the day shift tech had to come in at 3 a.m. This went on for some time until a night person could be hired. Staffing nightshift is not easy. Not only is it a difficult adjustment of biorhythms but night shift techs must be able to work independently. They are responsible for much of the maintenance of the machines. That can be extensive and can have serious ramifications on work output if it isn't done right.

Were there conflicts? Of course. Day shift would calibrate any new lot of reagent and clearly mark that it was new. That made it safe to use for patients after it was verified with controls but we all knew we must not start on the new lot until the old lot was gone. Woe be it to the tech who accidentally opened a box of the new reagent before the old lot was used up and failed to run the required controls and make notation in the action log. He or she would definitely hear about it from the senior tech on day shift. New boxes of reagent of any kind had to be dated and initialed when opened so there was no wriggling out of responsibility.

Second shift techs felt that day shift did not understand how busy we were and we sometimes resented it when we were criticized for some petty infringement. Day shift did not think we appreciated all they did in calibrating and keeping track of the control statistics as well as ordering.

Mistakes were also brought to our attention by day shift since it was those techs who examined any corrections made on the computer where results were stored. Not all results were automatically sent from the machine to the computer. There were still manual tests. If we had pressed the verify key and realized, too late, that we had misentered, we had to use the correction option and call the floor to tell them we had corrected. All dayshift had to do was pull the corrections sheet and our errors were there for all to see. I made a mistake myself in the early days when I failed to notice a zero value for a sugar. It was evidently a small bubble in the sample and for some reason the computer did not flag it as critical and I did not correct it. The senior tech from days pulled me aside and showed me the report. I was very embarrassed as the doctor had called and questioned it. She was kind and understanding but I never did it again.

It was a happy day for both shifts when we got autoverification. Our computer system was then able to release any result automatically without perusal by a tech so long as it was not critical and was within pre-agreed ranges. Very abnormal results still pended and were rechecked. My zero sugar would not have gone out with autoverification. We worried at first that this was not a good thing as we were used to seeing every value but we soon learned that, with our volume, the computer was better able to filter out the results that needed our attention and results went out faster to the doctor or to the floor.

During my time there, my hospital was judged as one of the 50 best hospitals in America and I felt it was deserved.

Interview with a Tech (2023)

Please tell us your name, shift and duties.

My name is Nikki Fulton. I work night shift at a medium size hospital. I have worked in the lab for 43 years. I immigrated from Greece when I was 14 years old. I spoke a little English as I had taken it in school but my teacher in Greece was from England so the American accent was hard for me to understand. The American culture was very different as my little community in Greece was very conservative. I went to work in a factory making chamois cloths, made from hides. The smell was so bad, it took my breath away. I was determined to make a better future for myself so I attended first St. Petersburg Community College and then went on to the University of South Florida. I then received my medical technologist license. My father paid for my first degree but when I moved on to USF, I had to take out loans, about $25,000 in total. I first worked in a reference lab on night shift. Then, I worked in a doctor's office lab on day shift while also working in a hospital lab at night. I worked nights for five years until my debt was paid.

What is the biggest challenge for you in your job? Are the hours or shifts a challenge?

I think new policies and regulations are challenging. They have a good purpose but it is an effort to keep up with requirements. New technologies are coming along all the time and we have to adapt to using them. I have worked various shifts over the years. I work nights now. When I am off for a few days and then go back to nights, it is tiring. I feel I didn't get enough sleep but when I get into the groove of night shift, it's better. Nights can be frantic but they are often quiet.

Is your job different since Covid? How did it affect you?

I was working in the main lab during Covid. It was very stressful. We were geared up all the time to get the work out. People were getting sick so sometimes I had to work double shifts to take up the slack. We had to be gloved and

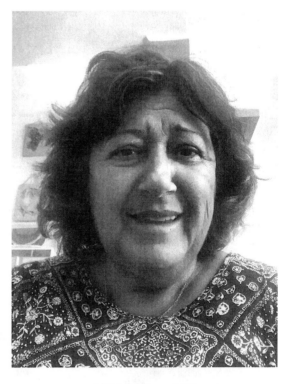

Nikki Fulton, MT

90

masked but I still got Covid myself. Then there was the emotional part, the worry that we wouldn't get results out in time and, of course, I was away from my family more than usual.

Do you feel stressed in your job?

I am not as stressed as I once was. After Covid, administration hired more people. Since we are better staffed, I only have to work every fourth weekend. That is important to me because I have a teenage son who wants to go places on weekends.

If you feel stressed, is support of any kind offered in your place of work?

My present supervisor is wonderful, very compassionate. My previous supervisor was also good. I started feeling ill one night during Covid. I tested myself and the test was positive. I called her and she told me to go home immediately. There was another tech on with me so the work still went out.

How does it affect your home life? Do you find it difficult to balance work and the rest of your life?

I have recently begun working three 12-hour shifts. I need to be at home as much as possible for my son. He is 16 and was running around unsupervised. I now work 7 p.m. until 7 a.m. three nights per week. He still would like to have me provide transportation in the evenings which I can't do every evening but at least now I can do it four evenings a week.

Do you feel recognized as part of the healthcare team?

Of course not! In the lab community, we are appreciated but the outside world has no clue. When discounts were being offered to first responders during Covid, lab techs did not qualify. Only doctors, nurses, firemen and police were included. But we were handling the infectious specimens every day. We were being infected ourselves but we still weren't considered important.

Do you feel satisfaction in your work?

Yes. I am helping people diagnose their problems. If I see a patient who has had a BUN of 5, then I see that the next BUN result on that patient is 30, I call the doctor to alert him or her to the change. I'm glad I went into the field. I can't imagine doing anything else. Techs are committed to their work.

Would you recommend young people go into this field? Why or why not? What would you tell them about the field?

Yes, if they like to be able to figure out disease states and help others, it is a satisfying feeling.

EIGHT

A New World:
The Microbiology Lab

Though I loved my team in chematology, I still longed to work in micro and I finally got the chance in the year 2000. It was again a second shift position. Cultures came in culturettes (small tubes with some nutrient solution to keep bacteria alive during transport) and in containers for urines and stools. I began on the set-up bench. I can't imagine that anyone would choose this particular bench on a long term basis as it involves taking the culturette and inoculating various culture plates from the sample, hundreds of them. Everything gets a blood agar plate as it will grow almost anything. A so-called chocolate plate (not chocolate but the color of it) is added for respiratory specimens and wounds and a MacConkey for gram negative organisms. There are other medias for stools and anaerobic specimens. Fortunately, the computer would spit out the proper number of barcodes for the type of culture ordered so it was a clue as to how many and which plates to use.

The volume was even greater than I had experienced in the main lab because we did all the microbiology for four of our system hospitals plus the outreach doctors and nursing homes. Nursing home patients are subject to several different stool pathogens because of proximity and poor resistance. Stool cultures required several different plates because so many conditions can be detected from the stool. Ordinary pathogens such as salmonella and shigella are found in stool but it is also cultured for campylobacter. People who eat raw oysters can develop one of the Vibrio species and it is detected in the stool. Serology tests are set up for clostridium difficile (C diff), a bacteria unfortunately found to be transmissible in the hospital or nursing home environment. We also set up wet preps for WBCs. There should be few if any WBCs in stool and a large number of them alerts the doctor to inflammation. Absence of bacteria in the stool is also a red flag as the bacteria in our gut are the workhorses in digestion and they also make some of our most important vitamins available for use by the body. If the bacteria are absent, probably due to antibiotic use, the doctor needs to be informed. Parasites could be found in stool and a stool for ova and parasites was often ordered with the culture.

This lab had a tube system that brought in samples from the floors. The tube was sealed and could be used for all samples except blood cultures which might have broken in transit. It made a clunking sound when the tube hit the bottom of the shoot and it became standard practice to call out "Incoming" when we heard that sound as it often meant stat work. On really busy nights, we groaned when we heard an incoming much as we groaned in the main lab when we heard the sirens from the ambulances as they brought patients into the ER. We weren't lazy and we were always aware that these people needed us but it was only human to find yourself overwhelmed with so much work and all of it time sensitive.

All the plates were necessary because certain organisms will only grow on the right plate at the right temperature. For instance, hemophilus, one of the bacteria responsible for meningitis, will only grow on a chocolate plate. A missed media plate might mean missing a pathogenic organism. If the bench tech realized that a plate was missing, there would be delay while the specimen was searched out later and inoculated on the additional plate.

I have never seen the sense in using technicians or technologists for setup duties because it does not require licensure but it did give me a good start in micro. We had many blood cultures as anytime bacteria get into the blood it is called septicemia and is very serious. They were carefully drawn after a three stage process of cleaning the patient's arm because you don't want to introduce any contaminants from the skin. There are always two bottles, one for aerobic bacteria and one for anaerobic since the circulation is a closed system and bacteria that do not require air can grow in the blood. The bottles are put into a machine to incubate, and the bottles are gently shaken. One night the shaking wasn't happening on one machine. There was a noise coming from the machine that wasn't moving. We thought, perhaps, something had rolled under the instrument so I got on my back on the (I'm sure) contaminated floor and starting peering up underneath with a flashlight to see if I could dislodge an offending item. At that moment, I remember thinking how useless all that chemistry and physiology were to me right then. We should have had Toolbox 101 where they would give us a little red toolbox and teach us how to use the contents. There were so many instances where we had to take something apart or put it back together.

After I had suffered the setup bench long enough, I started on the urine bench. The UTIs (urinary tract infections) are micro's bread and butter. Evening shift did not do the majority of the urine cultures. They must incubate a certain number of hours before you can be assured that they have had sufficient chance to grow. Second shift only worked up the ones that were set up too late for first shift to read. It was a good shift to begin to learn because there were fewer urine cultures than on days.

Once again, I had a great team. Hoamy, a Vietnamese-American tech patiently trained me in TB. Roland, of Mexican descent, taught me to use cumin as well as micro knowledge. A tech from Colombia, one of the kindest people I've ever known, remains dear. I was most fortunate in my primary trainer in micro: Mel Hauge was an older and very experienced tech who took me under his wing. Not only was he knowledgeable, he had a great sense of humor. He was from Minnesota and came in one evening looking like Hagar the Horrible with his Viking helmet on, complete with horns. Evidently, it was some special day in his home state. His favorite holiday was Valentine's Day and, on that day, he suggested we all write "I love you" in any language we knew. He wrote it in Norwegian, I wrote in English, Hoamy wrote in Vietnamese, Roland wrote in Spanish and we had a woman that evening from the Philippines who wrote in Tagalog. I still have that paper today.

With some experience, you get to know some organisms by appearance and smell. Staph and strep don't grow on MacConkey. Though they are both white, Staph bubbles when a small amount of peroxide is dropped on a colony. Strep doesn't. Pseudomonas smell like grapes. Klebsiella smells to me like dirty socks. E Coli has a sharp odor. They have different growth patterns. Proteus swarms and can cover the plate. Klebsiella is mucoid. For some types of bacteria, appearance and a few chemical tests were all that was needed to identify the organism but the rules are very specific. Many organisms (we called them orgs) had to be confirmed via panel. These were cards with microwells imbedded in them. Each well contained a chemical which would either change color or turbidity according to the org's specific reactions. We made suspensions, using enough colonies from the plate to conform to a standard. We had a turbidity meter to make sure we were within range as it was important to have enough org in the suspension to allow the reactions but not so much as to overwhelm them. When we set up an identity panel, we also set up a sensitivity panel to tell the doctor which antibiotic would be best to kill this org. The sensitivity panels were also cards with microwells of antibiotics. There were different panels for gram positive and for gram negative orgs as many antibiotics do not work on both. The cards had sipping straws attached and we put our tube of suspension on a machine called the Vitek with the straw inserted into the suspension. The machine would sip a specified amount into the card and read the reactions at the appropriate times.

A report would print out after some hours identifying the organism or, in the case of sensitivity panels, giving us a report on whether the org was resistant or sensitive to the different antibiotics. This was especially important in the case of staph. There are several kinds of staphylococcus but the one we most wanted to identify was *S. aureus*. The name aureus is from the Latin for golden because it is a yellowish color. One staph is resistant to the usual antibiotics, particularly methicillin, so is called MRSA, methicillin resistant staph aureus. At that time, most MRSA was found in hospitals and in nursing homes and patients with it were isolated to prevent spread. It is unfortunate that community acquired MRSA is prevalent now and is found all over. Efforts must be made all the time to find new antibiotics to combat not only MRSA but other resistant orgs. So many antibiotics are used in animal husbandry and even on crops that resistance is inevitable. One new idea is to use bacteriophages which are natural enemies of bacteria and, hopefully, will defeat the resistance problem. It was all a far cry from reading reactions in individual tubes as we had in the old days but Florida's population had increased by millions and we would never have been able to complete our work if we had not had the instrumentation. Of course, many cultures had multiple organisms and they had to be painstakingly isolated by subbing different looking colonies onto new plates and re-incubating.

I moved from urines to blood cultures. We were not using Bactecs at this time in my hospital but I have used them in other hospitals and the machines we had used a similar methodology. Bactec machines could detect growth by monitoring carbon dioxide production that occurs when bacteria grow in the bottles. In the Bactec bottles, there is a dye that fluoresces in the presence of CO_2 (Bactec, 2014). A light would go on and a jarring sound would alert us to the presence of a positive blood culture. There were different bottles for aerobic and anaerobic culture. We would take the positive bottle off the machine as soon as possible.

There was no chance of forgetting as the alarm went on until the bottle came off. Sometimes it was a contaminant from the skin and not a true infection but we gram stained a sample from every positive bottle and, if we saw bacteria, we had to call the floor if it was an inhouse patient, call the nursing home if it was a nursing home patient or call the doctor if the patient was neither. On the weekend, the latter took up a lot of time as we got an answering service and had to wait for the doctor to call us back. We then took a sample of the positive bottle and subbed it to the appropriate agars. Our lab had a dedicated anaerobic incubator, but in smaller places we had to seal the plates in a pouch and include a substance that took the oxygen out of the bag. We included a control strip to make sure the bag was indeed without air. Yeast can also grow in blood cultures and is a serious pathogen in people with compromised immune systems. We had panels to identify the types of yeast.

I used to dread getting cultures on homeless people. These poor folks live rough, with no opportunity for proper sanitation. When they finally show up in the ER, it is usually bad. They could have multiple organisms in their blood, urine or respiratory systems or in all of the above. Many are subject to substance abuse and poor nutrition and have low immunity. It seems that the money which is spent trying to cure these complicated conditions could be better spent on shelters and places for these folks to bathe and wash their clothes. Rarely have they applied for Medicaid so it all is charged to city or county entities and the hospital hopes they will get some reimbursement for the outlay.

We did not do respiratory or wound cultures on second shift but we had kit tests to use for diagnosing the different kinds of flu, stools for occult blood or any other kit not done in the main lab. One kit was especially important. Streptococcus, abbreviated strep, is initially identified by the hemolysis it produces on a blood agar plate. Hemolysis is the term we use for the breakdown of red blood cells. We use a lot of Greek letters in the lab and hemolysis is called beta, alpha or gamma. Beta hemolysis is characteristic of beta strep, strep pyogenes, which means fever producing. It is also called Group A strep and is the most common organism causing strep throat.

Group A almost totally lyses the red cells in the blood and creates a clear zone around the bacterial colony. Group A strep can be a serious pathogen because, if untreated, it can have sequelae including rheumatic fever affecting the heart or Bright's disease (glomerulonephritis) of the kidneys. Alpha strep creates a green hemolysis caused by incomplete breakdown of the red cells. Strep pneumo results in alpha hemolysis. Gamma is the term for no hemolysis at all.

Another important strep is Group B strep. We tested for this org particularly in expectant mothers or those who had just given birth because it can be passed to the baby in the birth canal and cause a type of pneumonia, septicemia or meningitis (CDC, Fast Facts, 2022). At that time, we were using a kit test for identification of Group B specimens coming from the OB unit or from local obstetricians. Those tests, plus the stats that came in during the evening including stat gram stains from the ER or emergency surgery, could keep one tech busy an entire shift.

Eventually, I began training in the TB room. Tuberculosis has been a scourge for centuries. We have all heard of patients dying from consumption, the term once used for the disease, because patients became very thin as the germ consumed their lungs. Whole families could be wiped out because it is contagious and people living together with an infected person are more likely to contract the germ. Robert Koch discovered the bacteria causing the disease in 1882 and was later awarded the Nobel prize (CDC, MMWR, 1982). In some parts of the world it is still called Koch's bacillus. For many years there was no good cure and patients were sent away to sanitariums both to give them the best conditions for cure and to keep them away from the general population.

Since the advent of AIDS, we have seen far more TB because of decreased resistance among the HIV positive people, among cancer patients who were receiving chemo and among people in poor living conditions. It has always been around. When I was a child, returning soldiers from Korea brought TB home with them. My adult cousin was one of them. I often went down to their farm as a young child and anyone who was thirsty while they were outside drank water from the pitcher pump in the barn lot, all using the same tin cup. I was exposed along with his children. The health department in Indiana came to realize that there was a mini-epidemic and they came into the schools and tested all of us. Eight children in my school tested positive, including me at age seven.

I went for chest Xrays yearly as a child along with the seven other kids in my small rural school to make sure we never developed the disease. I don't think any of us ever did. Just because you have the germ, it will not likely grow unless you become run down. Good nutrition and healthy living conditions often prevent the bacteria from taking hold but there is always a reservoir in the population, especially among the homeless and the immunocompromised. Tuberculosis is most often caused by Mycobacterium tuberculosis but I learned that Mycobacterium avium was also being found in patients with AIDS. We had a special machine for incubating TB cultures with bottles similar to the blood culture system and a negative pressure room for TB which did not allow any bacteria to escape to the rest of micro or outside to the environment.

A special stain is required to differentiate TB from other bacteria. We call it an acid fast stain and bacteria that are resistant to it are called AFB, acid fast bacilli. The procedure is to make a direct smear from a sputum or from a culture, then dry and fix the sample to the slide with heat. We then used Carbolfuchsin or a similar red dye, followed by a wash with acid alcohol. The last step used a methylene blue stain. Ordinary bacteria will take the blue stain but will not retain the red stain. Mycobacteria are resistant to the acid wash and stand out as narrow red rods among the blue components. Techs are expected to review one hundred fields under the oil immersion lens as there may be very few bacteria and you don't want to miss them. Few direct smears at our hospital were immediately positive but allowing the bacteria to grow in culture greatly enhanced the likelihood of detecting the disease.

Perhaps because of my history, I really liked working in the TB room and used that knowledge in the next phase of my career.

Interview with a Micro Tech (2023)

Please tell us your name, shift and duties.

My name is Roland Zapata. I work second shift in microbiology for a large hospital chain. I have worked in the lab for 28 years. I first earned a degree in biology but soon found that there were no jobs available using that degree. My sister was looking at a brochure and saw that my degree could be the basis for a degree as a medical technologist. I went back to school and trained as an MT at Texas A&M, Corpus Christi. My blood drawing experience was for only two days. The first day I watched the phlebotomist and the second day I was on my own to draw. I only drew three patients but I remember it well because one of the patients I observed being drawn was handcuffed to the bed! When I was a certified

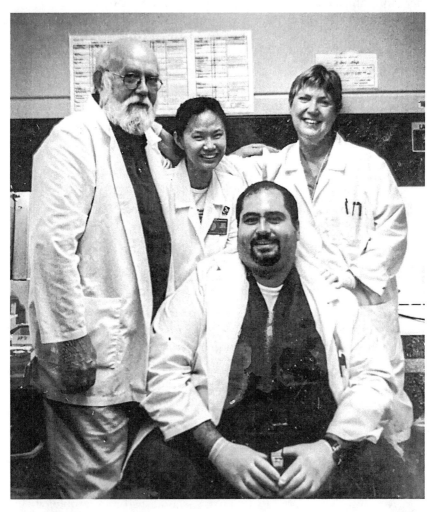

Standing, from left: Mal Hauge, MT, Hoamy Lin, MT, author. Seated: Roland Zapada, MT. Mal, sadly, has passed away.

technologist, we did go to the floors to administer and read PPD tests, the test to see if someone has been exposed to TB. Because I already had a science degree I was able to take the test for ASCP registry as soon as I finished my 18 months of training. I worked in hematology on second shift for only three months before a day shift position opened in micro and I have worked in micro or molecular ever since. I worked a second job for twelve years, three days a week and every third weekend in order to pay off my student loans. This was in addition to working every third weekend at my primary job.

What is the biggest challenge for you in your job? Is the shift a challenge?

I like second shift because there is time to get other things done during the day before I go to work and the shift diff is another reason. It isn't so great for a marriage if the other partner works days but we have persevered. The work is good but, since we are now doing all the micro for 16 entities, there is a lot of it. Also, personalities can be challenging. Some of the new people are enthusiastic about the field. The older techs aren't as enthusiastic as they once were. Changes in management, changes in procedure, changes in general take a toll. There are LMAs who are doing their training with us after completing a degree in science as I did and they are a big help. They make sure I have supplies and they help with setups.

Is your job different since Covid? How did it affect you?

Covid was unreal. During Covid, our referrals department refused to package the specimens going for sendout testing so, on top of all the testing we were already doing in micro, we added that duty to our workload. The minute I walked in, there was much work waiting. We immediately started running and we didn't stop. It took us about two weeks to get our flow. The number of tests was daunting and there were different methodologies depending on the order. Abbott came out with a rapid test but we were also running on the GeneXpert. There were multiple platforms to use but before we could even begin testing, the sample had to be processed. We set up under a biosafety hood using a face shield and other PPE. We had hooks mounted on the side of the biosafety hood and there were always eight to ten face shields hanging there because we each had our own. Of course, other tests had to be done in addition to Covid tests. We still had MRSA, Beta Strep, Cdiffs, urines for legionella and others as well as the endless Covid testing. We were burned out.

Do you feel stressed in your job?

It can be stressful. If we have an LMA to help, it isn't bad but sometimes we have to work without them. I no longer work any overtime and I gave up the second job after twelve years. I seem to be struggling to do it for the last year and a half. I guess I'm still burned out.

If you feel stressed, is support of any kind offered in your place of work?

(Laughing) I use cigars and rum. My grandparents came from Mexico. They had a real fire to better themselves and their families and I have noticed the same fire in other immigrants. I have to remember the sacrifices they made and I keep going.

How does it affect your home life?

When we worked different shifts, my wife and I didn't go out much. It was hard to spend time together.

Do you feel recognized as part of the healthcare team?

No. For example, the hospital puts up banners for Nurses Week or Doctors Week. They are prominently displayed. One year, they actually put up a banner for Lab Week in one of the main entrances to the hospital used by coworkers but it was only up for one day before it was relegated to the hallway that led to the main laboratory. We work behind the scenes but they need us whether they acknowledge it or not.

Do you feel satisfaction in your work? Are you glad that you went into this field?

Yes. I enjoy micro. Sometimes we find organisms that are new to us and they keep renaming the others so there is always learning. I know what we do is important though it may not be appreciated. I'm glad to have a fulfilling job and I am glad to have had the opportunity to go into it.

Would you recommend young people go into this field? Why or why not? What would you tell them about the field?

(He hesitates.) If they like the medical field and they don't want patient contact, I tell them to go for it. The pay is decent now though it can be stagnant. The increases are not much considering that we now do twice the amount of work that we used to do. We have to use speed to get it all done. And the administration seems to staff only the number of people to do the job as though no one will ever be off so, when someone does take off, we're working short. Of course, there are slower days, too, but I sometimes feel like the administration does not care about our concerns.

Interview with a
Special Chemistry Tech (2023)

Please tell us your name, shift and duties.

My name is Hoamy Lim. I work day shift in special chemistry. Our facility gets samples from all over our system of hospitals and doctors' offices. We do electrophoresis and immunoelectrophoresis as well as other assays to test for allergens and other autoimmune diseases. I have been a tech for twenty-five years. I came from Saigon, Vietnam, when I was four years old. I first attended a local community college in their medical technology program. I then worked in microbiology for three years and was able to earn my state medical technologist license. I had to pay for my education myself. I arranged my schedule so I could work fulltime as a nursing assistant while I was going to school. It wasn't easy. I did have loans but not too much.

What is the biggest challenge for you in your job? Is the shift a challenge?

I find the biggest challenge to be keeping up with new technology. New ways of testing come out all the time and we must learn them. There are also competencies and continued education modules to complete. I like day shift because I still have teenage children and it allows me to spend time with my family.

Is your job different since Covid? How did it affect you?

I was working in molecular during Covid which is outside the hospital. It took time to get geared up for all that testing but I don't think it was as bad for us as it was in the hospitals because we were using the Cobas 6800 and the BD Max and could test in larger batches. It was certainly busy but I did not do overtime. Our area was well staffed.

Do you feel stressed in your job?

Not so much in my department now. When I worked in molecular, it could be stressful because, if the QC (quality control specimens run with every batch) failed, everything had to be rerun which was hours of work. I didn't need any more stress in my life as my husband had a stroke and could not drive at the time so I was doing all the transport of my kids to their activities, to doctors' visits, etc. He walks and can drive now and that is a big help.

If you feel stressed, is support of any kind offered in your place of work?

My supervisors have been great. I was diagnosed with breast cancer when I was 47. It was another kind of tech who probably saved my life. I had gone for an ordinary screening mammogram but, when the mammogram tech asked me if I had any lumps, I admitted that I did. She refused to do the screening and insisted that I go back to the doctor and get an order for a diagnostic mammo. I was annoyed at the time because I had taken time off to get the mammogram done. But I did get the order and it was cancer. It was already in my lymph nodes. I had surgery, chemo and radiation. My place of employment allowed me to work part time during my treatment. I would get my chemo on a Friday so I would have the weekend to get over the side effects. Then I was able to go back to work on Monday.

How does it affect your home life?

I've been fortunate to have a supervisor who really listened and cared. My son had terrible eczema when he was little and the day care facilities did not want to take him because of the itching and rash. I was able to work part time, mostly weekends, so that I could be at home with him during the week. He is now a senior in high school. He still has eczema and we have to be very careful what foods he eats and what he is exposed to. It's frustrating because I can't do more to help him.

Do you feel recognized as part of the healthcare team?

Within the lab community, yes, but not in the outside world. People see my scrubs and still think I'm a nurse or a doctor. It's hard to explain what I do so that people understand.

Do you feel satisfaction in your work?

Yes, I enjoy what I do. This is a real profession and I am able to talk to other professionals and learn from them. This job has allowed me to take care of my family since I am the only one working.

Would you recommend young people go into this field? Why or why not? What would you tell them about the field?

Honestly, if they love the work and don't care about making lots of money, I'd say yes. But it doesn't pay as well as other fields. I will be forever grateful for the insurance benefits, but the insurance is expensive. New people have to go into it knowing that they won't get rich doing lab work.

NINE

Mission to Ethiopia: Setting Up a Lab in the Desert

In the year 2000, it suddenly occurred to me that, for the first time in my working life, I was supporting no one but myself. Both of my children had completed their educations and were on their own. It gave me a feeling of freedom. I remembered seeing a news clip in 1999, when Doctors Without Borders won the Nobel Peace Prize. I was full of admiration for what they did in the developing world and thought, at the time, what a great thing it would be to be able to volunteer. After my epiphany of freedom, I went to the website for Doctors Without Borders, which, in the rest of the world, is referred to as MSF—Médecins sans Frontières, French for Doctors Without Borders. It was a French group of doctors who began the charity in 1971 as a reaction to the war in Nigeria. They wanted to have an independent body of volunteers who would help in times of crisis anywhere there was a need without partiality. By the year 2000, from the three hundred volunteers who began the organization, MSF has grown to include 63,000 staff in seventy countries (Borders, 2022).

I was a little disappointed after reading the list of positions available in MSF, because lab techs were not mentioned. I went no farther in my application at the time but got to thinking about it later. If lab techs weren't needed, who was doing their bloodwork or micro? I knew it couldn't be doctors or nurses because they don't receive lengthy training for that sort of thing, at least not in this country. Of course, lab staffers are used to working behind the scenes. I thought maybe I should look behind the scene on the MSF website, too. I clicked on present needs and what popped up but lab techs!

I made out the application right then. It included my educational history and experience. After some time, I received a call to come for an interview in New York. This was at my own expense but I really wanted to do it. I had lived in Brooklyn for a few months when I was 19 but that had been more than thirty years ago. This time I stayed in an older hotel that was still expensive. I was baffled by how to handle the cage around the elevator until the owner came to my rescue by pulling the accordion door closed so that the elevator could actually move. I remember that the hotel description promised a continental breakfast. That turned out to be a chit that I could take across the street to the coffee shop for coffee and a donut.

The staff at MSF, New York, could not have been nicer. It turned out that they had been looking for a lab tech for a long time. I suggested that they make that need a little clearer on the website. Later, I came to realize that the main reason MSF had trouble getting lab techs in this country is because they want a commitment of at least six months. Very few lab techs can get time off from their jobs for that long, nor could many pay their bills while they were away, though MSF does give volunteers some money while they are on mission, which is paid into their account at home. In my case it was about $600/month in 2001. Had I been obliged to pay a mortgage on that, I could not have gone on mission but I had downsized enough to get by for a period of time. My primary contact was a woman from Liberia named Hawah. She explained how everything worked and asked me questions about what I expected and what I was willing to do.

My application went out to the teams in the field and I later received a call from a doctor in Paris. She explained that MSF USA operates in league with MSF France. There were positions in Turkmenistan and Uzbekistan, but the most pressing need was in a TB mission in Ethiopia. She cautioned me that the place in Ethiopia was quite hot. Oh, well, I thought, I'm from Florida. I can do heat. She told me that, because they did not have a tech, the staff were forced to send sputum specimens to a hospital many miles away. The specimens were drying out in transit and the team did not feel they were getting accurate results. I knew I could do TB work and she assured me that, though this mission was under the auspices of MSF France, it was an English speaking mission and all team members would be able to speak my language. I took the job.

I did not ask for six months off. I knew better than to expect it. I tendered my resignation with an explanation of what I was going to do. People were surprised to say the least. I had been told to get as many of the required vaccinations as possible before I left and I also had to get a test for HIV. I was able to get the vaccines for yellow fever and for hepatitis A from our local health department but I hit a stumbling block when I asked to have the HIV test at the hospital. The tech refused to draw and run it without a doctor's order. Of course, she was within her rights since we are supposed to have an order, so I went downstairs to the pathologist I knew best. I asked if he was familiar with the group Doctors Without Borders and he certainly was. I explained that I was going to go on mission with them and needed the test. He marched upstairs with me and gave the order to draw the test. The result was negative and I was ready to go.

About five weeks before my departure, I met a man on a birding trip and we had several dates before I left. He seemed to be a great guy but I never expected him to wait around while I took a job in Africa

In May of 2001, I once again flew to New York with a large suitcase. I took a hair dryer, a few dressy clothes, multiple pairs of shoes, cosmetics and other assorted paraphernalia. Hawah helped me schlep this suitcase down the street to the van which would take me to the airport. The one smart thing I did was to buy a Foder's guide book to Ethiopia though I had yet to read it.

The plane was late arriving in Paris. I had to negotiate getting that big suitcase up elevators and down corridors at the airport with the signs in a language I did not understand until I found the van that would take me to the MSF headquarters. Since I was late, I had already missed an appointment with one person. While I waited for my next appointment, I met a logistician who had just returned from my mission in Galah. From him, I got the real story. The only electricity would be from a generator which was only used when necessary and from solar panels that powered some lights at night. So, there was no reason to take that hairdryer. He went on to tell me that I would be in a tent and my clothes would be washed for me by having native people scrub them on a washboard. It was clear that I wasn't going to need those dressy clothes or the cosmetics either. I got permission to store the suitcase in a closet at the headquarters and was given a duffle to contain my severely whittled down possessions.

I met with different people that day, first with a counselor who advised me on behavior while on mission. She told me not to do anything to embarrass my country and not to do anything that would embarrass MSF. She warned me about hand gestures with the explanation that they might not mean the same thing to others that they did in my culture. I next met with a nurse who began the rest of the inoculations that MSF requires volunteers to have. I got the first of my rabies vaccines. The second dose was to be given before I left for mission and the third went with me in a cooler to be given after I got there. I was vaccinated for typhoid and for meningitis, the kind caused by *Neisseria meningitidis*. This was years before this vaccine became available in the U.S.

Lastly, I was told about my particular mission but I really didn't get much out of the briefing because I was going to sleep from jet lag. The only thing she said that stuck with me was the line "Your team will sustain you." Truer words were never spoken.

On the second day, I met with Lawrence, the female doctor who had called me. She checked me on finding the TB bacilli in a slide which was easy for me but I did not do so well on the malaria slide so she coached me on that. Then, for a couple of days, I was free to walk around Paris. There was a holiday in France during my time there and I also had to wait to get the second rabies shot. My hotel was basic but pleasant and paid for by MSF. There were no elevators. People there climb stairs. There was a lovely room on the top story where we had breakfast: baguettes, croissants and fruit. I had been to Paris as a tourist but I noticed this time that shop owners were nicer to me. Parisians are tired of tourists and can be abrupt but, if I wore the MSF T-shirt that I had been given, it was a different story. The French people are very proud of MSF as they have a right to be.

I left Paris on May 24 and, hours later, I landed in Addis Ababa at night. I had been told that there would be someone there to pick me up but people who are not traveling are not allowed to hang around the airport there as they do in the States. In the dark, I couldn't see anyone waiting for me. I had also been told that, if someone was not waiting, to take a taxi to the MSF guest house and not to pay them more than $10.00 American. This was not so easy as I was besieged by taxi drivers who had only rudimentary English. I found one who said he knew where the guest house was and so began a long slog through Addis because he really had no idea. Finally, he stopped at a pharmacy where he got some directions. I wound up at the MSF Belgium guest house but the person in charge of their division kindly drove me to the proper one for MSF France. Needless to say, I was very tired. I had expected heat but it was cool and the very thick double woven blanket on the guest house bed felt good indeed.

Addis has a great climate. I saw many plants that grow in Florida but also some that grow farther north. The highlands of Ethiopia are fertile and it seems that enough food could be grown to feed the people but the infrastructure is lacking. The wife of the head of mission in Addis came to the guest house and took me to buy food for the few days I would be there. Veronique was a doctor herself, an obstetrician, but she was not allowed to work in Ethiopia because they had a rule that, if one person of an expat couple was working, the other was not allowed to work. What a shame this was when the country, at the time, had a high maternal death rate. My head was on a continual swivel as we drove through the streets with the open-air markets spilling out onto the streets and the herds of goats being driven down the traffic lanes. There was a man whose legs had been blown off during the war with Eritrea. Men were expected to fight but there was no social service to take care of them when they returned after being wounded. This man's torso sat on a skateboard and he rolled out to beg when traffic slowed down. Veronique said she gave them whatever change she had. She could not give more because there are too many of them.

The headquarters for all of MSF in Ethiopia is in Addis. It was within walking distance and I walked down there to pick out the kits I would need for mission. The kits are a marvel of organization. There were kits for obstetrics, for surgery, for therapeutic feeding, etc., but I was most concerned with the lab kit. The worker there opened it to show me the microscope, slides, slide box, stains, gloves, masks, pipettes, cotton, everything I could need in one box. This system is the reason MSF can have a whole field hospital up and running within a few days of a disaster. Tents and medical supplies are also boxed so it is just a matter of pulling the right boxes off the shelf.

I had lunch with the workers at the headquarters. The cost was fifty cents. There are several tribes in Ethiopia. Mostly people of the Amhar tribe live in Addis and their food staple is injera, a flat pancake made with a grain called teff. Onto this base, they pile fillings, spicy lentils, potatoes and rice and vegetables. It was quite good.

At the headquarters, I was able to read my email and to let them know that I had arrived safely. It was a nice surprise to hear from the man I had met just three weeks before leaving. He was a birder like me and he was eager to hear about any new birds I saw.

When all was packed, I left for a mission. There were three of us in the cab of a small Toyota pickup, the driver, myself and an Italian

American doctor who would be volunteering in the hospital some hours from our mission. It was an eight-hour drive and the farther east we went, the drier the landscape became. We arrived at Galah in the late afternoon and I was introduced to my team. Maria, a Greek nurse, was head of mission. We had two doctors, Milton, a Quebecois doctor who had founded the mission, and Vinod, from Australia. There were two logisticians, abbreviated as "logs," who did everything nonmedical. The French log was responsible for ordering and general maintenance while the other, Jose, who was originally Portuguese but naturalized French, was involved in building living quarters to get us out of the tents.

The landscape was so different from that found in Addis, it was hard to believe that I was in the same country. We had come through the mountains on our way and I could still see them in the far distance but everything around me was flat and gray. I had arrived in the Danakil depression, also known as the Afar Triangle. This area, in the northeast corner of Ethiopia, is part of the Rift Valley, once wet and verdant and home to one of our ancestors, the famed Lucy, discovered in 1974 and named *Australopithecus afarensis* after the area (Hurum, n.d.) but now the land was sunken to as much as four hundred feet below sea level (Willock, 1974). The soil is gray dust because the area is volcanic. There is a phrase I heard later referring to the inhospitable nature of the region and attributed to an Eritrean, "Even a jackal makes his will before he crosses the Danakil." It's just as well I hadn't heard that before I arrived.

About half a mile from our tents there was a strip of green created by the Awash River. Dr. Milton founded the mission here because the population had been noncompliant in completing their TB treatment when they were treated in the city. The Afar people survive on goat milk and meat and they couldn't take care of their animals in the city. Here, the women wove mats from the reeds growing beside the river. Then they took pliant branches from the acacia trees and bent them into arching trusses which they covered with the mats. In this structure, whole families lived, often three generations of a family.

The team had better success with sustained treatment in this location. The only thing they had been lacking was a lab technician to read the slides. Anticipating the arrival of said technician, they had built a laboratory, the only solid structure in mission. I could see it from our living area, a block building with windows on all sides. Our living compound consisted of tents for the five of us expats, a larger structure for our native staff, including interpreters and native nurses, a dining hut and kitchen and a wooden office on stilts. There was a loosely woven fence between us and the hospital tents.

I had done a lot of camping so it wasn't a problem to sleep in a tent but I didn't sleep well due to continual coughing from the hospital tents just beyond the fence. In addition to the TB patients, they had an outbreak of whooping cough. Whooping cough is caused by a bacteria, *Bordetella pertussis*, and was very rare in the States at the time though it has made a resurgence now due to the fact that not everyone gets their children vaccinated. Because the Afar people are among the most stoic on Earth, they often did not report symptoms until the disease was beyond the point where antibiotics would help very much. So the treatment was basically supportive, including IVs to rehydrate them since they coughed so violently they vomited and couldn't drink enough. Then, to add to the noise, there were the hyenas, a sound I wouldn't call a laugh. I lay there wondering what on earth was making that sound and finally got an answer from the team the next morning.

The next day, we went up to the lab. It was obvious that a lot of effort had been put into getting the new lab ready. There was no running water in the living quarters but, here, they had built a platform and hefted a large plastic drum onto it filled with clean water. This allowed us to have a steady supply of water in our lab. This was a necessity for rinsing slides. There were benches on both sides with large windows. This was important as our microscopes were set up to use mirrors that would reflect the sunlight coming through the window onto the stage of the scope. There were light bulbs included in our kit but no electricity to run them. A new cabinet was ready for the supplies I had brought with me and a kerosene powered refrigerator was installed.

Next, we visited the hospital tents. It was strange to see patients lying on mats on the ground but with IVs running. But it was a real hospital with a chart system in place and a clinic area out front for seeing outpatients. I spent the day in the lab getting set up. There was a balance in my lab kit which made it possible for me to weigh the crystals and dilute the stains necessary for staining AFB. Somehow, though I had read slides with Lawrence, it had not really sunk in that these slides were the only way we had for actually detecting TB. They were so seldom positive at home even in patients who would later have positive cultures, that I was afraid we would miss cases. Cultures were not possible and the kit tests available now had not been invented. But I set up my slide boxes for retaining slides after reading just as we would at home. And I cleaned. It is essential that any lab be kept clean but especially so if you are dealing with bacteria. I knew, if we had positive cases, bacteria could waft into the air while making slides from the sputum specimens and could contaminate the air or other slides. I asked for bleach and was informed that the Afar had been taught to call it Javel water, a term used for bleach in French Canada. After I used the right term, I was given some bleach which I diluted and used to wipe down everything. We were ready.

By afternoon, I realized what hot really meant. It was 110°F every day and some days it would be hotter. The sand burned my feet through my sandals. Maria made sure I got my "gourd" which was not a gourd but, rather, a cleaned plastic oil bottle which had a burlap covering. The idea was to fill the gourd and then dip this burlap covering into water with the assumption that the evaporation would cool it. She showed me the filter system where all of us expats needed to get our drinking water since we had no immunity to the organisms of this new environment. And she warned me to drink, drink, drink. Dehydration was a real danger.

In the morning we were given tea in our dining hut, which was open in the front. Tiny weaver birds had made nests in the ceiling. We sat on mats that the Afar women had woven. They were paid for their labor by MSF as were the men working on the crew quarters under construction. MSF also paid for native nurses and interpreters. We ate a type of dense bread which was unfamiliar, but it was good and filling. Water had to be hauled from a wetter place far away when I got there and sometimes the log would bring back oranges from that site. Lunch was always rice with some veggies mixed in. It was tasty but dinner was always spaghetti and it wasn't. Italian food is popular in Ethiopia because the Italians took over the country in 1935 and stayed until they were ousted in 1941. The starchy pasta every night got old for all of us.

I began patient care by watching the doctors in clinic. They asked me to do hemoglobins and we had a clever device for doing that. It was handheld, with a wheel on one side and two glass plates on the other. The wheel had colored inserts correlating to levels of hemoglobin. I pricked a patient's finger and the blood ran between the two glass plates in a thin film. I then turned the wheel until the shade of red on the wheel matched the color density of the patient's blood film and read off the number from the wheel. Everyone was anemic, usually about eight grams. Their diet of milk and bread did not supply enough iron and I was to learn that many also had parasites including malaria.

Though it wasn't mosquito season yet, my team all began taking Larium, a preventative which does not keep you from getting malaria but does keep you from getting cerebral malaria which is often deadly. I had no problem with it nor did Maria but the men had terrible dreams bordering on hallucinations and had to be switched to a different med. Fred, our log, either did not take his preventative or he missed some doses because he contracted malaria when he went for water in the wet area of the Triangle. I walked into our living compound and saw him lying on the porch of the office, wrapped in heavy blankets in the godawful heat and shivering.

I had mixed my Geimsa stain, the gold standard for malaria stains, as instructed by Lawrence, but it did not work. Perhaps it was because the pH of the water was wrong. Even using the distilled water from my kit did not help. Distilled water bottled in some plastic bottles does not stay at a neutral pH. If the plastic is permeable, it can allow gas from the air to alter the acidity in the bottle even before it is opened. For whatever reason, I was not able to find the parasites in Fred's blood. Malaria parasites have a growth period and the shivering only starts when they have matured in the red blood cells and rupture into the blood. Fred was treated anyway but I vowed to get a better handle on my malaria stain as the wetter season was coming. Over time, I found that I could see the tiny rings of *Plasmodium falciparum* in the cells using ordinary Wright stain such as we used for differentials in CBCs.

The Afar people were well aware of TB which they called thin man's disease in their language. Indeed, the patients were thin and it was easy to see why it used to be called consumption. They knew it killed. My new helper, named Hammadou, brought the first sputums up to the lab the next morning. I had been asked to train some Afar young men to read for TB and malaria. The lab had been built to WHO standards, with an anteroom which could be shut off from the main lab while we were smearing the sputa on to slides, drying and staining. This was a learning experience for both of us. He had to learn to wear a mask , though I'm not sure he understood the reason for it. I had been told to just run a flame under the slide after it was dry to fix the specimen to the slide, then to flood the slide with the individual Ziehl-Neelsen stains.

We were supposed to run the flame under the first fuchsin stain to facilitate the uptake of the stain but the stain was drying far too fast on the slide in this step, bubbling in the heat and forming crystals. I had a kerosene refrigerator in the anteroom and the thermometer on it read 38°C which is about 100°F at 6 a.m. Between the fixation step and the ambient temp, the slides were just too hot. When I looked at them under the scope, there were crystals everywhere, occluding any possible organisms. I had to find a new way. Fortunately, I had filter paper in my kit, for use in filtering the stains. I found that, if I cut a slide sized piece of the filter paper and laid it over the dried and fixed slide before we added the stain, the stain would "take" before it got too hot. The next slides, using this method, were much better and I needn't have worried that I would miss cases through lack of culture methods, because many slides were positive for TB. When I did my statistics before leaving the mission, I had a positivity rate of 26 percent on direct stain, a rate unheard of where I worked in the U.S.

My helper did not know any English beyond "good morning." Lawrence had shown me, in Paris, how to teach without language. I had a blue ink pen and a red pencil. I drew a circle on paper with the background cells in blue and the thin rods of TB in red, just as they appeared in the microscope field. It took several days and several drawings, but one day we had a eureka moment when he suddenly realized what he was looking for. After that, I only needed to train him to quantify as 1+ 2+ 3+ or 4+. Thank goodness we both used Arabic numerals.

We began work at 6 a.m. to take advantage of the relatively cooler mornings. We would only have the sun at the proper angle to fall on the mirrors for about two hours in the morning and two hours in the afternoon so we tried to get the slides ready as early as possible in order to start the microscopic examinations. The Afar broke at 11 a.m. and did not work again until about 4 p.m. It was understandable since the heat was enervating to say the least. Anyway, we could not read without sun for our microscopes and it was not available through the windows when it was high in the sky. During this break, my assistant went down to the hospital tents if he was needed there or he rested.

I made up stain, cleaned or otherwise busied myself, but, after sitting in the window in the sun for hours, I was broiling. I could sit in the dining hut after lunch but it wasn't much cooler. Some people slept during the break since we got up so early but my tent was much too hot. It seemed like wasted time. When the sun had sunk to the proper location, we returned to the lab. There were bench high counters running along both walls of the lab and the routine we developed was to stain all the slides, using our masks in the anteroom, then to read as many as possible in the morning before we lost our light, then to return to the lab in the afternoon, move the microscopes to the opposite side of the lab to catch the sun on that side and finish reading on that side until we once again lost the light in the late afternoon.

We had a satellite phone and were allowed to send emails once per week. I would compose my emails to family and friends ahead of time and send them quickly on the appointed day. I could download my mail at that time, too. The connection to home was much appreciated. Maria was very careful about satellite phone use, however, because it was expensive. We had a radio and most communication with Addis was done via radio contact. Of course, there was no cell phone service. I also wrote letters and they were mailed when someone went to Addis. I didn't want to take too much satellite phone time telling about the birds and animals I was seeing when I went down to the river after leaving the lab in the evening but it was worth telling in a letter. African birds are colorful and the tiny antelopes called dikdiks and the warthogs were worth mentioning. Guinea birds and Marabou storks ran around outside the lab and I could see the Afar men moving their camel herds to greener areas from the lab windows.

When I first arrived at mission, MSF staff were doing all the cooking for the patient population and their families. It was a labor-intensive operation since food was cooked on wood fires on the ground in steamy conditions. One day, we had a bucket brigade of medical and native staff, handing out food to an increasingly large number of people. Maria said "This has to stop. This is not what we should be doing with our time." Supplies were ordered to hand out to the individual families for making their own food. When they arrived, she checked every plastic plate and utensil as well as the food stuffs to make sure it matched the packing list. She kept a close eye on MSF assets and was a great head of mission at only 26 years old.

This mission was having much better compliance from patients since they could keep their goat and camel herds nearby. The protocol at the time was for two months in the hospital tents while receiving four different drugs for TB treatment followed by four more months of coming to the DOTS (directly observed treatments) tent daily for two of the same drugs. It was vitally important to keep the patients from wandering away before completing treatment because, if the TB germ was not dead, it would develop resistance to the drugs being used and make it much more difficult and more expensive to continue treatment later as MDR (multi drug resistant) TB. Milton had situated the mission near the river as the greenery there was something for the goats and camels to eat. The reeds growing there were also used for the ubiquitous mats.

While I had never seen anything other than respiratory TB in the States, I saw my first two cases of TB of the spine, commonly called Potts disease in mission. One was found in an old man and the other in a young girl. The disease had caused her spine to bend and it was one of the great successes of our mission when I saw her before leaving with a straight spine.

The TB germ can survive stomach acid and swallowing it could lead to disease of other organs. When I was a child on the farm, we drank raw milk but I remember pasteurization being discussed. I remember that my mother thought it was a good thing because many people had dairy cows back then and she said TB could be passed in the cow's milk as well as other bacteria. That AFB is *Mycobacterium bovis* and it can cause havoc in multiple organs systems. When I see unpasteurized milk being sold now, I remember that. The cows are probably tested regularly but why take a chance?

One young girl had TB of the kidney. She was a beautiful child and I was glad she was getting help. In fact, many of the Afar women were beautiful. The Afar had long been mixing with Arabic and European peoples over the centuries because of their nomadic lifestyle and it showed in the faces of the women. They were slender and small boned and it was easy to see why they might have problems with childbirth. Added to that, the Afar practiced the most severe form of FGM (female genital mutilation). While a little girl was still very small, a woman of the tribe would cut away the labia and the clitoris and sew the outer lips closed so that only a small opening was left for urination and menstruation. It was an abhorrent practice and our doctors as well as the native nurses were doing their best to stop the tradition.

Milton had been successful in stopping one young mother from circumcising her last two girls after the first one had been sewn so tightly that she could not urinate and almost died. Glad as we were to hear this, I wondered what effect it would have on the girls' future, since Afar men might not consider them "clean" enough for marriage since they were intact. I asked our liaison if the practice was decreed in the Koran but he said "absolutely not." He said that the custom had begun with the pharaohs in Egypt centuries ago and had nothing to do with religion.

I have said that the Afar were a stoic people and the women had to be particularly so since I was told that the husband was expected to "break through" on the wedding night and I can't imagine that the opening was large enough to easily accommodate intercourse. Other sources indicate that the new husband will cut that area on his wife on the wedding night in order to accommodate intimacy. Either way sounds terrible. For childbirth, the stitching was cut but in some cases the woman is sewn up again after the birth (UNFPA, 2022). This practice, plus the delicacy of the bone structure of many of the women resulted in fistulas, the rupture, during difficult labors, of the vagina into the rectum, causing enormous suffering. Feces and urine could leak from the vagina. The women smelled and could be ostracized.

Valerie Browning, a nurse/midwife from Australia, had come to the area to help, and formed, with her brother, the Barbara May Foundation. She worked mostly with the Afar and her brother, a surgeon, repaired fistulas on women from other regions of Ethiopia. I never met Valerie but she had influenced Milton when he was establishing this mission. I am happy to know that her organization is still functioning today and has even built a small maternity hospital in a nearby village (Foundation, 2023).

One of my first challenges in the lab was the flies. From growing up on an Indiana farm, I knew that livestock draws flies. We had cattle, goats and camels in mission and the flies were everywhere. Our food was brought to us with a cover over it but the minute the cover was removed, the flies attacked. It was frustrating in the dining room, but in the lab, it was dangerous. There were no screens on the windows which we needed to keep open because of the heat but the sputum specimens attracted the flies and, possibly we did, too, since our bodies were always coated in sweat. If a fly landed on a positive sputum specimen while it was being used to make slides, then flew on to another slide or onto the counters, it could spread the TB germ on its legs. One of my first requests was for screens which had to be ordered from Addis but the team did everything they could to accommodate and screens were procured. We had no frames so Jose taped them to the windows and it did a lot to keep the flies out.

Flies also led to trachoma of the eyes. The disease is caused by the bacteria, *Chlamydia trachomatis*, and it was spread by the flies which were attracted to the fluid in the eye. The bacteria irritated the eyelids so much that the lashes turned inward and scratched the cornea which could lead to blindness. Vinod showed me a middle-aged woman who had suffered with this disease for years and was almost completely sightless. What a shame, when it could easily have been treated early on with some antibiotic salve and basic hygiene. The same bacteria can live in the genital tract and cause disease. It is one of the reasons why babies get eye drops after birth to avoid infection obtained in the birth canal.

Vinod showed me my first case of Madura foot, technically called Mycetoma. Madura foot is a fungal condition found in tropical countries. Vinod had seen the condition in immigrants to Australia. It results in awful draining sinuses with purulent discharge. It begins when there is a wound to the foot and the fungus finds its way in. It can get so bad that excision and debridement become necessary. Fortunately, this patient did not require extensive surgery but I was reminded why our presence there was important because without treatment, the condition would have worsened.

The Afar, being Sufi Muslims, did not work on Friday, their Sabbath. The rest of us still worked seven days a week and, for that and other reasons, the expats among our team were encouraged to travel to Addis every six weeks for R&R. Milton had ended his time in mission so we were down to one doctor and one day, while Vinod was in Addis, a young pregnant woman was brought in. Maria examined her, which she would have had to do, even had the doctor been around, because the Afar men would not allow male doctors to examine their wives or daughters internally except in rare circumstances. Maria ordered a urinalysis and I found 4+ protein in the woman's urine which indicated, along with the high blood pressure readings and her symptoms, a condition called preeclampsia. It is life threatening and the only treatment available was delivery. The woman had to be transported seven hours to a hospital where they did an emergency caesarian. I was told that, though she had been in a very painful labor for many hours and the ride over rough country was exceedingly bumpy, she had not made a sound during the long journey. Thankfully, she delivered a living child. Had we not been there, she would almost certainly have died.

So much of lab work in the U.S. is what I call "cover your butt" medicine, where the doctor orders tests, not necessarily because the patient needs them, but, rather, so that there can be no questions asked about lack of testing in any future lawsuit. It was truly refreshing to know everything we did was absolutely necessary. And I felt every bit a part of the medical team at mission. The lab was not sequestered as it would be in the States. I talked directly to the doctors and nurses and I felt I contributed a necessary skill which was recognized because it was visible.

Maria woke me one night to tell me that a child had been brought in with suspected meningitis. They wanted me to do a gram stain of the spinal fluid. Of course, I would have been happy to do that, but I had no sun and therefore, no microscope. It was decided right then that we had to find a better way to light the scopes. The next morning Jose wired our scopes to a solar panel outside the lab, inserted the light bulbs that had come with our kit and voila, we had artificial light. To be certain that any organisms will be seen in a spinal fluid, the fluid should be spun in a high speed centrifuge but all we had was a hand cranked system. My trainees could crank a lot harder than I could but it still wasn't fast enough to get much of a sediment. I need not have been concerned. I put a small drop of the spinal fluid on a slide, gram stained it and found *Strep pneumoniae*, often called Pneumococcus, all through the fluid and the child was suitably treated. Later, Jose rigged up a battery attached to the solar panel so we could store power and use it at night. Better yet, we could read slides all through the morning and afternoon, without sitting in the windows in the blazing sun. This was a great improvement as the heat was merciless. At one time, I felt my trainee gently reach over and wipe the sweat off my forehead before it fell on the microscope. The solar panel meant we were still dependent on solar energy but there was never any lack of sun.

I had moved on to other trainees during my time at mission. The next three were much easier to teach because Hammadou stayed on to explain things to them in their language. They were bright and willing and I thought it was a shame that they could not go on to train as healthcare workers. This wasn't likely as all higher education in Addis was given in English. The Afar speak French as their second language if they have one and they were therefore excluded from jobs which they could well have done had they had access to training. Most of our native nurses spoke English as well as French and Afaric and served as interpreters as well as performing medical duties.

Another great improvement in mission was when the French contingent of the NGO, Action Against Hunger, dug a well for us. No more carrying water in huge bladders from distant places. Because of the volcanic activity under our feet, the water came hot out of the ground. The children ran into the spray as the pump started up and we got into the spirit, too, letting it wet us all over as a welcome relief from the heat. They then piped it to a central location and we did not have to be so sparing of water use after that. Fred even started a small garden to grow some melons since he now had water to irrigate it.

Oscar was an eight month old infant brought in due to failure to thrive. I examined his mother's sputum the next morning and it was full of TB. Tuberculosis can be passed in breast milk so both mother and baby had to be treated. Maria also put the baby on a therapeutic feeding program and, when I left three months later, he did not look like the same child. Our little miracle.

HIV was not a big problem in mission but it was huge in Addis. I read that 70 percent of the "bar girls" in Addis were HIV positive. One man came to mission from Addis, supposedly to work with me, but it soon became apparent that he was a patient instead. The HIV testing kits MSF had planned for me to keep on hand could not be used because our refrigerator, which worked well in more temperate climates, could not keep reagents at the required temperature in the intense heat. Even without laboratory diagnosis, when our new arrival took off the warmer clothing he had arrived in, it was obvious that he was far from well. At the time, there was no good treatment for AIDS available there and we were not equipped to treat it. This man was finally taken back to Addis to seek treatment there. But the team was aware that the disease was only a matter of hours away and we were concerned that, by paying the men to work on the living quarters, it was giving them money to go to other cities, to visit prostitutes, and possibly to bring HIV home with them. With so many already weakened by TB and malnutrition, they would not have had much resistance to HIV.

Poor nutrition was exacerbated by parasite infection. Despite Maria's heroic attempts to get our two kitchen girls to change the dish water and to use soap and a little bleach, we often saw the morning dishes at lunchtime, still soaking in cold water with no visible suds. Add the fact that they seldom washed their hands and it is easy to understand why Maria and I both picked up Giardia within the first months I was there. Giardia is a one-celled parasite. It is found in the States in freshwater rivers and streams that have been contaminated with human or animal waste and is the main reason why trekkers have to use a water filter or chemical to avoid it. Though we had plenty of metronidazole, which kills it, we knew treatment, under the circumstances, would be useless. One day, she caught the kitchen girl filling our canteens with water straight from the old bladders rather than from the filter system. We would have been promptly reinfected. Instead, we spent a lot of time rushing to our one toilet. Jose had created an outbuilding of sorts away from our tents. He poured a sloping cement floor with drains. He then put up a framework around it and wrapped it in mats. One side was our shower where we dumped a five gallon bucket of water over our heads and on the other was our primitive type toilet which was just a hole over which you had to squat. I began to lose weight, not a bad thing in my case but the diarrhea sapped what energy I had that wasn't already sapped by heat.

Another parasite we had to watch for was Schistosomiasis, or, as the natives called it, Bilharzia. It could be picked up by bathing in the river, which the team was warned not to do but which the Afar did regularly as it was their method of getting clean. The protist (one-celled organism) could crawl up the urethra and block the exit of urine. It was said to be extremely painful. The laboratory manual that I had been given in Paris said to spin the urine down by using the centrifuge but I didn't have much faith in our hand-cranked version. The manual was written in French but it was surprising how much I could understand by looking at the pictures and diagrams and I could always get someone to interpret if necessary. Fortunately, I was never asked to look for that parasite but I did learn, from the Addis tech who replaced me, that the proper way to do it is to use a beaker of some kind (he said they used old light bulbs with the end cut off), and set it in the sun. The parasites come to the light and you can simply set a slide on top and they will adhere.

I did discover *Entamoeba histolytica* in a patient's stool which was very exciting for me as I had seen the cysts in the U.S. but had never seen the living trophozoite. I remembered having learned that it moved in only one direction unlike Entamoeba coli which moves erratically. I ran down to the hospital and asked Vinod if he had ever seen it since I knew it was seldom seen in the West. It may seem strange, or perhaps unfeeling, that we would find pleasure in someone else's illness but it was a scientific discovery, not schadenfreude.

I had heard about sand storms in the desert but I got to experience one for myself when huge dark clouds blackened the sky one day while I was cleaning the office during our break. The wind picked up and we were warned by native staff to get inside. Maria and I sat back to back in the office with the shutters closed as much as possible. The whole building shook and the sun was completely blotted out. It was scary and it did a lot of damage, including to our tents.

I went to Addis for my break after about two months. I was not feeling well but still managed to go to the museum to see Lucy. What tourists see is actually a reproduction as the real Lucy stays below in the proper conditions to preserve her. I also went to the foreign market and bought food for my team as they always bought for the rest of us when they went to Addis. I bought peanut butter which was appreciated by all, Afar and expat alike. I also bought shredded coconut which I used to make a kind of ambrosia concoction using oranges that the logs had bought during my absence. It was a big hit and all the native staff as well as the imported folks crowded into the dining hut to try it out.

To my dismay, my second trainee, a very pleasant young man named Adais, had waited until I returned to tell me that he wasn't feeling well. His eyes had the glassy look of fever. When I touched his forehead he was burning up. Before I even told the doctor, I pricked his finger and Gram stained the slide for malaria. Many red blood cells included ring forms with the two red dots of *Plasmodium falciparum*. When I trained, back in the 60s, my mnemonic for learning the types of malaria included "falciparum is fatal." It was fatal in 1968 but, thankfully, we had the treatment now and he was treated immediately. I was so sorry that he had continued working, while he was sick, waiting for me to stain a slide. I made up my mind right then to teach these young men to stain and detect malaria as well as TB.

Malaria is endemic in many parts of the world but not all of those areas are home to falciparum. According to WHO, the most vulnerable group are children aged five and below. In 2021, 95 percent of malarial deaths occurred in Africa (WHO, 2022). It is spread by the bite of Anopheles mosquitoes. The organism travels in the blood to the liver, which is the reservoir. It then matures in the red blood cells as merozoites, which we call ring forms, since they exist as tiny rings inside the cell. When the cell is full of parasites, it is called a schizont. This cell ruptures and spills the tiny organisms into the blood. This is when the patient feels the chills, the body's response to this foreign invader. Different types of malaria have different maturation cycles but all we saw at mission was falciparum. The danger with this type of malaria is that, untreated, it will attack the nervous system and, indeed, we had a young TB patient who did not report her malaria symptoms when she came to the DOT's tent and was too far gone when she was finally brought in by relatives. We all grieved when she died as it was unnecessary.

Improvements were happening when I returned. Since we no longer needed to sit in the sun to read our slides, I had permission to buy fabric for curtains while I was in Addis. Headquarters sent a man to drive me and to do the haggling. This was a great blessing as the mercado was a rabbit warren to me and I would never have found all the components necessary. Fabric was at one shop, thread at another and curtain rings and rods at yet another. I cut and hemmed the fabric when I returned and the rods were hung so we could shut out the brilliant light during the hottest part of the day. That dropped the temp a few degrees. The permanent living quarters were still under construction, but Jose and his helpers had built temporary sheds for us with gravel floors and mat dividers since the tents had been destroyed by the storm. It was more comfortable than the tents and we really appreciated how fast Jose had got them done. Maria, Karen, who was our new French nurse, and I slept in one shelter and the men in another.

August was the beginning of the rainy season and we knew there would be an upsurge in malaria cases. I wanted to be ready but, at the same time, I felt weaker every day. Not only did I have intermittent diarrhea, but I also had heat rash all over my arms and torso which only responded to antihistamines if I took so many that I was wobbling on my lab stool. One day, I had to return to my shelter and lie down before my work was done. I woke to find both Vinod and Maria crouching over me, caring for me instead of our patients. I asked Vinod what he thought I should do and he said he thought I should go home. It was a painful decision as these people had become very dear to me but I did not want to be a burden. A replacement tech was found in Addis until a tech from MSF could come from France. He spoke English well and was the one who told me how to use the light bulb beaker to find schistosoma. In talking about his training, I found that he had used the same books for his training that I had used earlier in my career. Once again, I wished that my trainees could have had access to this training, but there was the language barrier. I also knew that they might not have wanted to leave their desert home and people. It was hot and mostly barren but it was home to them.

I left mission in early September of 2001. I was in the New York office of MSF just one week before the World Trade Centers came down. After that happened, I received, via email, a wonderful letter from the team at mission, including the Afar members, expressing sorrow for the horror and asking after my welfare. The Afar members of the team were all Muslim, but they did not hold with terrorism.

I looked at my surroundings in my Florida town with new eyes, seeing for the first time the waste of plastic bags and bottles used so indiscriminately and tossed when they would have been treasured finds for the Afar people at mission. I was changed physically, having lost 18 pounds, and mentally, having seen my culture from the other side of the mirror.

Doctors Without Borders needs techs. In countries with a national healthcare system, my team members coming from those countries told me it was possible to take whatever time they needed for a mission and still be assured that there would be a position for them when they returned home. In our system, a tech who might want to go on mission would have to either negotiate time off without pay or quit entirely as I did. I wrote an article for *Clinical Laboratory Medicine*, the magazine published by the ASCP, describing my experience in mission and I hope it encouraged other techs to go as it is a most fulfilling experience. Later, I wrote a book about my experience. Doctors Without Borders systematically gets four stars from Charity Navigator. I hope people are encouraged by my story to give to them.

Doctors Without Borders Today

On their website MSF describes itself as:

"An international, independent medical humanitarian organisation Médecins Sans Frontières (MSF) translates to Doctors Without Borders. We provide medical assistance to people affected by conflict, epidemics, disasters, or exclusion from healthcare. Our teams are made up of tens of thousands of health professionals, logistic and administrative staff—bound together by our charter. Our actions are guided by medical ethics and the principles of impartiality, independence and neutrality. We are a non-profit, self-governed, member-based organisation.

MSF was founded in 1971 in Paris by a group of journalists and doctors. Today, we are a worldwide movement of nearly 63,000 people (MSF, 2023).

On the same website, Doctors Without Borders lists the issues they confront:

"**Abortion:** Unsafe abortion is still one of the leading causes of maternal death worldwide.

Access to Medicines: Due to proprietary patents, many medicines are out of financial reach for much of the world.

Antibiotic Resistance: In countries without regulation of access to antibiotics, patients buy medicines over the counter which may not be the right treatment for their condition and which may cause resistance to bacterial infection in them and in the general population.

Cholera: 143,000 deaths per year.

Covid 19: The epidemic has taxed the resources of all countries but has been especially hard on those without sufficient medical infrastructure.

Ebola: Partially thanks to the efforts of MSF, the Ugandan Ministry of Health reported in January of 2023 the end of the most recent outbreak of this deadly disease.

HIV/AIDS: This is still a scourge with nearly five hundred children newly infected every day.

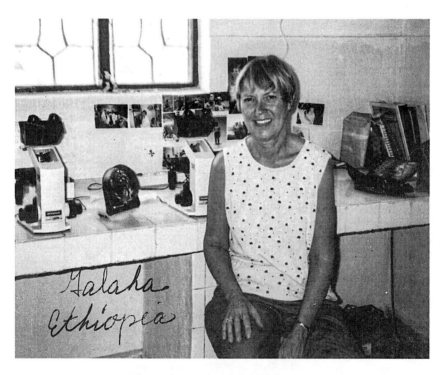

The author in her lab in Ethiopia.

Kala azar (visceral Leishmniasis): This parasitic disease is second only to malaria in numbers killed every year.

Malaria: Responsible for nearly half a million deaths every year with 70% of them children under the age of five.

Malnutrition: 232 million children worldwide are affected and malnutrition is a contributing factor in death from other diseases.

Maternal Health: 99% of women who die in childbirth are in developing countries.

Measles: This disease is still a leading killer, mainly due to lack of access to the effective vaccine.

Meningitis: The vast majority of cases are in Africa, including Ethiopia. Without treatment, up to half of patients die.

Mental Health: People who live in conflict and amongst disease need mental and psychosocial support.

Monkey Pox: WHO declared Monkey Pox a Public Health Emergency of International Concern after an unprecedented outbreak in number of cases in 2022.

Obstetric Fistulas: Often due to female genital mutilation and inadequate care during childbirth.

Sleeping Sickness (Trypanosomiasis): The disease attacks the central nervous system and without treatment is fatal.

Snakebite: Snakebite kills 20,000 people every year in sub–Saharan Africa.

Tuberculosis: Still the leading infectious disease in the world.

Vaccination: MSF gave out 3,200,100 vaccine doses in 2022.

Yellow fever: Many millions of people in Africa are at risk. A vaccine is available but without treatment, there is no cure."

TEN

Return to American Medicine

It was great to see my fellow techs when I walked into my former lab soon after returning home. There were many hugs and exclamations of surprise when they saw me so much thinner, with my hair bleached so much lighter and my skin burned so much darker.

There were no openings in micro at the time but I was fortunate that they took me back in the main lab. I was once again on second shift with my old comrades. My experience in mission was not wasted. One night we got an order for a malaria smear from the ER. I had done many of these in the U.S. in the past and they were almost always negative but one look down the barrel of the microscope and I knew it was P. falciparum. The two tiny dots on the ring inside the red cell had become familiar to me by now. We had a teaching microscope in hematology with two heads so that two people could look at the same view. I called my fellow tech over to take a look and he concurred. I called the senior pathologist, and he hurried up to confirm my diagnosis from the slide. He then went down to the ER and later told us that this sample was from a young woman who had gone to Africa as part of an aid mission and had not continued to take her malaria preventative for two more weeks after she returned per protocol. Fortunately, the disease was caught early and we all felt good about that.

The lab was busier than ever. Florida was and continues to be the fastest growing state in the U.S. and our area was home to many elderly. Age brings ailments and having Medicare assures that people of that age or older are entitled to treatment at no or little cost to them. I am grateful for Medicare but, perhaps because I had just returned from a no cost treatment facility, I often felt it was not entirely fair for older people to have such a great benefit when we had young Mexican families wander into the lab with sick chicken in tow, speaking no English, trying to find the ER. Often, they were forced to use the ER for any medical problem because their jobs did not provide health benefits nor paid sick time. When these patients inadvertently found the lab, the only one of us who had taken Spanish in school had to try to communicate and he did so with a pronounced Alabama accent. Most times, he just led them to the ER where the cost for treatment would be far higher than it would have been at a regular doctor's office or even at a walk-in clinic.

These people were not beggars. They worked and probably paid into social security and Medicare, though it might have been under an assumed name if they were not in the U.S. legally. They would not be able to collect that social security or Medicare when the time came because they would not be able to come up with the required birth certificate in the name they had used to pay in. Although it may not be fair to the taxpayers who could wind up covering the medical care of illegal immigrants through tax outlay to the hospital, it is a fault of the system. Statistics show that about 25 percent of documented aliens (non-citizens but in this country legally) and about 46 percent of the ones who are illegals are not covered by health insurance. Not only do their employers not offer them insurance, they are also not eligible for Medicaid or CHIP (children's health insurance) because they are not citizens. They face language and literacy issues as well (KFF, 2022).

Should we refuse care to these working people? They do not choose to get sick. I do not believe that the medical system would be overwhelmed if we had a national healthcare system. Any doctor will tell you that the myriad insurance companies with all their different computer systems require far too many clerks to do the filing and to refile if the company does not pay the claim, which is often the case. The proper diagnosis code must be used that will allow coverage of any test. Coders are in great demand, adding yet another employee layer to our already clunky system. A one payer system can work.

Though the systems in other countries may have problems, we should be able to learn from their mistakes and create something workable here. The KFF, formerly Kaiser Foundation, among other sources, reports that the U.S. spends far more per person on healthcare than any other country but has a lower life expectancy than Australia, Japan, and most of Western Europe (Rakshit, 2023). All of these countries have a national healthcare system. I have heard people say that they do not want so called "socialized medicine" because they don't want to pay for people who don't have insurance. Of course, they are already paying for those people because the hospital will collect from the county or the state for indigent care. They never get enough to cover all of it but what they do get comes out of your taxes.

Another factor driving up the cost of healthcare is the U.S. was the OSHA mandate for use of personal protective equipment. The law had been in effect for some time but it was an ongoing struggle for lab managers to figure out exactly what they were supposed to require and provide. Of course, we needed more safeguards than we had in the old days (which were none) but the new requirements could be cumbersome. Each tech changed gloves several times every shift. Our lab coats were supposed to be fluid impermeable and could not be put in the ordinary wash nor were we allowed to take them home and wash them. We had a service that took the old coats aways and we got a fresh one every week or more often if we got visibly contaminated. We were not supposed to wear our lab coats out of the lab. If we went to the cafeteria, the coat had to be left within the contaminated area. We had face shields to use when opening tubes because of the aerosol produced when the vacuum was breached or when working on tabletop instruments because tubing might pop loose and spray chemicals into our eyes. All of these things cost money.

There were other safety protocols. We had to wear closed toed shoes because fluid might fall on our feet if we were to drop something or dribble when transferring serum or reagent. Counters had to be wiped down at the end of every shift with freshly prepared beach. Since bleach does not retain its potency indefinitely, the bleach dilution bottle had to be dated and initialed to guarantee freshness. Everything had to be dated and initialed when the bottle or box was opened. The lab was required to do safety training on all new employees, and we all had to do periodic review of the safety systems and sign a paper saying we had done so. We had an eyewash station in case some tech got a chemical or patient sample in their eyes and a safety shower which I never saw used but it had to be tested regularly and delay ready for inspection. My friend, Elaine, tells me about checking the safety shower in her lab on the day before a JAHCO inspection. They turned it on and couldn't turn it off. It not only flooded the lab floor, it ran out into the hall and she had to work late sucking up the water with a vet vac.

In addition to the OSHA mandates, we had to participate in continuing education. The state of Florida required that we do one hour of continuing education units (CEUS) for every specialty in which we were licensed. I was licensed in six specialties so that was six hours every year in the specific departments licensed. There were required CEUs to be done yearly in medical errors and in HIV, one hour for each. The rest of the required 25 hours of CEUS could be in any of the laboratory disciplines. It was good to keep up with new developments but it took time. Administration made online courses available to us and I was able to do some of them while on the job but most of us had to do the majority of continuing education courses on our own time. Gone were the good old days when we could go to conferences, often sponsored by medical supply companies, and enjoy the camaraderie of other techs and the opportunity to learn from them. Cutbacks in Medicare had occurred plus there were now laws specifying what gifts companies were allowed to give to doctors and laboratories as incentives to use their services. Kickbacks to doctors and some private labs were notorious in some areas of Florida and the laws were needed but laboratorians lost access to an avenue allowing them to see and hear how things were done in other places with other procedures and instruments.

All of these state requirements had to be met if we were to be able to renew our licenses. Not all states require licenses for techs. Some accept national registry which I already had but Florida requires licensure and it is not free. My license was in six specialties and cost over $200 every other year.

Most laboratories employ a processing department. This is where the hundreds of samples come in from the many couriers we paid to pick up specimens from the various doctors and nursing homes that used our lab. We also had draw stations in various locations. Now, most computer systems in draw stations are so advanced that patient data are entered and barcodes print out when the sample is collected. Blood is spun down at the collection point when necessary for tests requiring serum. All specimens are put into biohazard bags and sealed for transport. At the time of my employment, most doctors' offices did not have the set up for barcoding so data entry had to be done in processing. We then had several processors who were not techs who entered data and separated the specimens according to which machine would be running them. Many tubes had to be split between machines. The barcodes were specific for the instrument. If a hematology barcode was accidentally put on a chemistry tube, the machine would not run it. Processing was particularly crucial on second shift since that is when the couriers came in so the majority of specimens were run on second shift. Specimen integrity had to be paramount and technical waited on processing.

Day shift might not have had the volume but they had much else to do. In addition to calibrating new reagents, they accompanied the doctors when doing bone marrow aspirations and they handled QC. This was a big job as everything was covered by quality control. Even the small cards used to do stool for occult blood had positive and negative controls. These results were logged. Positive and negative control slides were used to check the efficacy of the hematology stains. Not only were charts of all chemistry and hematology controls examined and evaluated by first shift, that shift was also responsible for the CAP (College of American Pathologists) surveys. These were quality checks required to get CAP certification of the lab.

Samples of unknowns were sent to be run in all departments and transparencies of cells and various organisms had to be examined by all techs that worked those departments. We all gave opinions on what the pictures displayed but our findings were confidential so we couldn't be influenced by someone else's opinion. We ran the unknowns on all shifts, and day shift collated the info and filled out the survey forms. It was very important to get these surveys right. If you got the same analyte wrong on successive surveys, the lab could be banned from running that test until you proved that the problem was corrected and that could take months.

In addition to QC, we had to run correlations every time we got a new instrument or new method of any kind. Though it was usually an improvement over the old method, certifying agencies, whether CLIA, CAP or JCHAO, involved doing what we called duplicate studies for correlation purposes. Patient tubes were first run on the old instrument, then we picked out the tubes with values in the low, moderate and high range and ran those patients on the new machine. We did this for one hundred values. The mean and SD (standard deviation) were calculated to make sure that the instruments correlated. If we found that the new machine and new reagents did not fully correlate with the old method, new normal values had to be instituted for the new method. That involved running one thousand normal patients and calculating the statistics on those values. The new values had to be entered into the computer systema and we also warned doctors that there were changes. It was a lot of work but every laboratory that accepts Medicare must choose a certifying agency. CAP is strictly for the lab. JCHAO inspects the whole hospital.

Maintenance of the machines was mandatory and done on third

shift when the machines were likely to be less busy. Tubing or probes had to be changed and cleaning procedures carried out. Even then, they were still running stat tests as all machines had backup of some kind.

After my return, I learned that one of our ancillary staff had contracted what was then called NonA NonB hepatitis. Hepatitis is a serious disease because it can lead to liver cancer in addition to jaundice, general illness and, in some cases, death. Hepatitis A is spread via contaminated food or water, is fairly common, and is usually short-lived. There is a vaccine for Hepatitis A. Hepatitis B was well known, even in the 1970s, to be a risk when handling blood and body fluids. A vaccine is also available for it. But, through time, it was recognized that there was a third kind of hepatitis, also present in blood and body fluids. Eventually, it was called Hepatitis C but it took thirty years before it could be definitely identified. It was understood that it was neither of the then known hepatitis viruses, but the specific cause was not isolated until 1990. And it was discovered, not by the traditional method of culturing, but by the new methodology of PCR.

Michael Houghton received the Nobel prize for his work in finding the virus but he freely admitted that it was the work of his staff, in particular Qui-Lim Choo who had done the bulk of the work, working seven days a week to find the cause (Ledford, 2000). A reliable test was finally developed to identify the antibodies in a patient's blood (Houghton, 2019). Our employee was lucky. She responded to the interferon being used in those days and was apparently cured. Fortunately, there are better treatments now for Hep C but there is still no vaccine. It was a reminder for all of us how important it was to follow safety procedures because we were handling samples loaded with all kinds of Hepatitis and HIV every day.

HIV was declining in the U.S. by 2001 due to better education and safer sexual practices. But we still often saw the ramifications of the disease in the lab.

We have previously talked about lymphocytes but they are especially important in the explanation of AIDS. This is a simplified explanation as the immune system is complicated. B lymphocytes are a type of white cell formed in the bone marrow and are responsible for the production of antibodies. Antibodies do not kill bacteria or viruses themselves. Instead, they "tag" invaders for the macrophages, the clean-up crew, to eliminate. T lymphocytes go through the thymus gland and are involved in recognizing cells that have been infected with a virus.

We have many more T cells than B cells. T cells are subdivided into subgroups. It is the killer T cells which destroy virus infected cells by releasing cytokines (Sompayrac, 2012). Helper T cells are memory cells. They remember a bacteria or virus that they have been previously exposed to and will activate the B cells to release antibodies to that specific invader. The system works very well normally but, in HIV, the virus inserts its own DNA into the host cell and hides there. It can remain dormant for a long time and continue to multiply while the immune system does not recognize the threat. HIV kills memory T cells. It is impossible to tell on an ordinary blood smear whether lymphocytes are B or T as they look the same on a slide but we did see lower lymphocyte counts in HIV patients. We also saw anemia in HIV patients and often low platelet counts (thrombocytopenia). More telling conditions would be diagnosed in the microbiology lab.

In addition to being able to survive undetected, HIV also has the ability to mutate so that, even if a T cell can recognize the first incarnation of the virus and kill it, it will not recognize the mutated version or the many mutated versions that follow. We began to send out a CD4 count, done by flow cytometry, as we did not have the capacity to run them inhouse at the time. CD4 is a protein that the virus binds to when it attacks helper T cells. The virus then either kills the memory helper T cell or makes it a target for the killer T cells since they will see that it is virus infected. In this way, HIV defeats the immune system because there will be no memory cells left to tell the killer cells to attack or the B lymphocytes to make antibodies to the many pathogens which can attack the immunocompromised patient. By keeping track of how many CD4 cells are present in the patient's blood, the progress of the disease can be ascertained as the CD4 count falls as more and more of the T memory cells succumb. Viral load studies are also used to monitor the disease (Sompayrac, 2012).

By this time, many people knew someone affected by this terrible disease. Thankfully, much better treatments have been developed that prolong life in these patients but it remains a concern for those handling the specimens.

Five of us manned the second shift. There was no evening supervisor but all of us were mature and experienced techs who were well qualified to recognize abnormal cells or results that needed to be questioned. Our laboratory computer system flagged critical results and they were not autoverified. The tech on duty had to repeat the result unless it was in keeping with a very recent value on the same patient. Critical values were always called. This could be time consuming in the case of an outpatient, as the offices were closed by the time we ran the specimen so we had to contact the answering service and wait for a call back from the physician. Notations had to be made in Cerner as to who had taken the result and at what time. It was a great team. And it was not the only good team during my career. I can honestly say that, over a period of over 40 years, I only remember three techs whose hearts were not in their work. They did the minimum. All the others, dozens of techs who worked with me, were truly dedicated and put everything they had into reporting fast and accurate results.

We were all cross trained in all departments and were regularly rotated so it was all familiar. One tech was kept busy running the cell counter and coagulation instruments. Although the machine could discriminate the types of cells, if there was any indication of an abnormality, e.g.: low red counts, white counts, platelets or a flag indicating unusual white cells, that sample had to have a slide made and stained, which was then examined by the second tech using the microscope. We took turns going to dinner so it was quite busy when you were in that department alone.

Our instrument for special chemistry was a Centaur from Siemens. It was an immunoassay analyzer used for quantitative pregnancy tests, tumor markers such as CEA or CA 19–9 which are specific for certain tumors, Vitamins such as B12 and Folate, antibodies to various diseases including hepatitis antibodies, PSA (prostate specific antigen), Ferritin (the storage form of iron), hormones such as FSH (follicle stimulating hormone) and LH (luteinizing hormone) and some of the cardiac enzymes. One of the most common tests was for the thyroid hormones. T4 (thyroxin), the most prevalent hormone made by the thyroid but the amount of circulating T4 is controlled by TSH (thyroid simulating hormone) which is produced in the pituitary gland in the skull. If the TSH is high but the T4 is low, that means the thyroid itself is not responding properly to stimulation. These tests can also be used to monitor treatment with replacement thyroid hormone. Special chemistry was also responsible for the many kit tests including the basic drug screens, qualitative pregnancy tests, etc.

It was not a matter of just putting the tube on the machine and walking away. The tech in charge had to constantly watch his or her pending list for the sample which perhaps had a clot or was too lipemic or had results beyond the linear range of the assay. Those samples had to be examined, diluted and/or rerun. On our shift, these samples were most often from the ER. All ER specimens were stat. Pregnancy tests were especially important because we were aware that a possibly a pregnant woman was waiting in the ER. The doctors did not want to do any further work on her until they knew if the patient was pregnant and, if so, how far along. Another patient might be waiting to know whether he had indigestion or a myocardial infarct. Stat samples were marked with a special sticker and had to be put on first. We really had to have our wits about us at all times.

Much of special chemistry was run on day shift since second shift handled the largest volume. HIVs were done on day shift. Along with immunodeficiency disease, there were the autoimmune diseases which had to be diagnosed and monitored. Autoimmune diseases occur when the immune system begins to see self as foreign. Lupus erythematosus is an autoimmune disease which affects about 250,000 people in the U.S., 90 percent of which are women (Sompayrac, 2012). You may have seen the "butterfly rash" across the cheeks which some patients exhibit. That is only an outward manifestation as the disease can also damage the kidneys, lungs and nervous system. In my early days in the lab, we did LE preps to attempt to diagnose this disease. The LE prep was a complicated and not very specific test for the disease. Later, we ran antinuclear antibody (ANA) tests which were much better though certainly not as good as the methods available today. Though many people who have positive ANAs do not have Lupus, almost all Lupus patients will have positive ANAs.

Another autoimmune condition is rheumatoid arthritis. It is a more serious disease than osteo arthritis since it often attacks younger people and is more debilitating. In RA, antibodies attack the cartilage of the joints. The reason why lymphocytes make antibodies against normal body tissue is unknown but IgM as well as IgG antibodies are found in the joints of people with the disease. These antibodies trigger the invasion of macrocytes and inflammation of the joint is the result (Sompayrac, 2012). There is a simple kit test for Rheumatoid factor but it's not definitive by itself. Other tests measure inflammation such as CRP (C reactive protein), and ESR (erythrocyte sedimentation rate). In a sedimentation rate, when whole blood is drawn up into a tube with gradations, the red cells fall faster when inflammation is present.

In multiple sclerosis, another autoimmune condition, there is chronic inflammation caused by T cells, which can cross the blood brain barrier, attack the myelin sheath around the spinal column leading to paralysis and sensory problems. It has been found that these T cells recognize the myelin protein but they also recognize the protein of the Epstein Barr virus, the virus responsible for mononucleosis (Sompayrac, 2012). Most people who get Epstein Barr do not get multiple sclerosis. The disease is known to be familial so it may be a combination of genetic predisposition and infection with the virus. No single test could diagnose MS at the time but there are antibody tests, many of which required sending out to an esoteric lab back then. The results of those tests, along with physical findings were used to diagnose.

A lesser known autoimmune disease is Sjogren syndrome. A dear friend of mine was diagnosed by her dentist due to the lack of saliva he saw in her mouth. The lack of saliva results in more dental cavities. Extremely dry eyes is also a symptom and fatigue is common to all of the autoimmune diseases. Sjogren is diagnosed with ANA but also with anti–SSA and anti–SSB as well as on clinical findings (ARUP, 2022). Don't assume you have Sjogren, however, just because your eyes are dry. Dry eyes seem to come with age.

The measuring of immunoglobulins has become more important in the diagnosis and monitoring of viral disease. IgM is the first response antibody with IgG following and lasting longer. My pneumonic for learning the sequence was to remember priMary. It is important to monitor the sequence of antibody formation in infectious diseases. The kit tests we use to find out if we have Covid or flu can pick up both IgM and IgG antibodies but, if we want to find out whether an infection is recent or of longer duration, we need to differentiate between those antibodies. Those tests can be done in the lab. Another antibody form we measure is IgE, which is elevated in allergic reactions. We often tested for antibody levels in patients who had contracted Lyme disease or Epstein Barr since both of these diseases can have lingering forms and doctors tried to judge whether there was improvement by ordering the different antibody levels.

Unlike Type 2 diabetes, usually found in middle aged or older adults and often linked to lifestyle, Type 1 diabetes is an autoimmune disease wherein autoantibodies destroy the insulin producing cells in the pancreas. The trigger is unknown. There are more autoimmune diseases, far more than I have mentioned, and it appears that they are increasing in frequency around the world. Some of the increase is due to better diagnosis but autoimmune diseases are cropping up in countries where they have not been seen before (Reed, 2022). Changes in diet have been mentioned and we are exposed to so many chemicals that were not present in the environment when I was young.

Maybe We Need to Use the Lab More Wisely

During my career I noticed that the most frequent reason for excess testing was the tendency of doctors to order the same test another doctor has already ordered on the same patient at a similar time. New computer control functions have made this less likely but simply not examining the chart to see what has already been ordered still results in duplicate tests. Another factor is the use of standard batteries of tests without regard to patient need. Below is an excerpt from a study done by the NIH on superfluous testing (Koch, Nov).

"Testing is an important part of medicine across all specialties and settings. As a result, the volume of testing is enormous, with an estimated 4–5 billion tests performed in the United States each year. Unnecessary laboratory testing and diagnostic imaging is believed to be common. Studies looking at testing of patients have found 40%–60% of tests to be unnecessary. Unnecessary tests can cause patient discomfort, patient harm, and increase healthcare costs.

"Interestingly, frontline physicians reported similar results as reviewers that the majority of patients had at least one unnecessary test ordered, and around one-third of all tests were unnecessary.

"We found that most patients experience unnecessary testing on the first day of an inpatient hospital stay. Around one-third of all tests were unnecessary by physician chart review. The most frequent types of unnecessary tests were laboratory tests. Beyond tests that were unnecessary by clinical guidelines, many appropriate tests did not change clinical care. Over the entire sample, 72% of patients did not have their care changed by testing.

"There were multiple reasons for unnecessary testing. Tests were often ordered as part of a triage protocol initiated when a patient was first seen in the Emergency Department."

ELEVEN

Microbiology Expanded

Though I loved the main lab, micro had my heart. It was like planting a garden without knowing what kind of seed you were putting into the ground. When you streaked that plate with a urine, respiratory or blood sample, it was the next day before you found out what org, if any, was in your garden.

A small hospital close to my home had a micro position open. It paid $2.00 an hour more than the hospital where I had been working. It always seemed unfortunate to me that the only way to get more money was to move to another facility but that was too often how it was. A coworker once described techs and hospitals as a dozen trees with a hundred monkeys jumping from tree to tree. The analogy was apropos as every lab I went to had someone I had worked with before who had resorted to changing jobs to get a raise. I never understood it as it must cost more money to hire and train a new person, who was paid more at time of hiring, than to give the extra money to the tech already working, but I saw it happen over and over.

This smaller hospital was a good place to work. The other techs were friendly, there was less stress and it was day shift. It was an ethnic community with its own culture which was fun to learn about. In the native language, the letter C was rarely used. Instead, we had a lot of names beginning with K. The carry-in dinners were fun as people there brought in dolmades and homemade baklava. I continued to work at this hospital part time even after I started drawing social security and will always cherish the time I spent there and the friends I made.

I wanted day shift at this time because the guy whom I had met before leaving for mission had stuck around and I married Merle Hubbard in 2003. I wanted to have the evenings with my new husband so the timing was good.

When I retired, there was a limit on the amount I could make in a year before they started taking part or all of my Social Security away. That rule has become less restrictive now. This is fortunate, since I had to turn down techs who wanted to take time off because, if I worked for them, I would be over the limit. After I reached full retirement age, the rule no longer applied and I found that I needed to work more than the hours I was getting at the smaller hospital. I went back to the large hospital on day shift, this time in micro and worked there until my final retirement.

We had a lab aide on day shift to do setups which freed the techs for the other departments. The benches were blood cultures, urine cultures, wound cultures, respiratory cultures, virology, mycology, TB, PCR and miscellaneous. My only disappointment in returning to this micro department was that the day of the white lab coat, symbol of our profession, was over. We now had blue paper coats, which must have been fluid impermeable per OSHA law because they were so hot. We simply threw them away when they got dirty and I suppose it was cheaper for the hospital than paying a service to wash them.

The miscellaneous bench was responsible for screening tests for flu, stools for occult blood or stools for WBCs and a special test using the blood of horseshoe crabs that detected the tiniest amounts of bacteria in the sterile water used for dialysis. This test, the Limulus Amebocyte Lysate test, LAL, was developed to detect bacteria in vaccines and even to test fluids sent to the space station. At Woods Hole, Frederick Bang tried to infect horseshoe crabs with bacteria and discovered that their immune system could surround the bacteria and form a gel around it, walling it off (Collins, 2017). The discovery led to using the blood for medical purposes. We did culture the dialysis water using a special filter but, since it was imperative that no bacteria be missed, we performed the LAL also. It was infrequent but, when bacteria were present, a small clot would form in the tube at the end of a many step process. It was particularly gratifying when culture and LAL agreed.

I worked again on the blood culture bench but found it to be a much busier bench than we had experienced on second shift. Many of the culture bottles were put on the machine in the evening so they had a chance to grow and turn positive on day shift. There were hundreds of bottles on the machines at any one time. They were kept incubating for five days so as to give any slow growing organism a chance to grow. The aggravating sound given off in the presence of a positive was far more frequent on day shift and there were times I wanted to scream for it to stop. I was working up the plates from the previous day's blood cultures, several cans of them, and it required concentration since some of them had multiple organisms and had to be subbed to isolate the different orgs. Panels had to be set up for identification and sensitivity and every loud alarm meant being interrupted. It was a day full of hear the alarm, take the bottle off, gram stain, plate, call the doctor, then, think "where was I on yesterday's plates when all that started?"

Every patient is given a unique multidigit number when he or she is admitted. We relied on these numbers as patients can often have the same name. One day a call came from the nursery asking for blood culture results on a newborn. She gave me the name and I could not find it in the computer. There were accusations of us having lost the specimens which I did not believe. The nurse insisted that the specimen was drawn. When she finally called back with the accession number, I was able to discover that the baby had been renamed. The mother had at first given the child the last name of the father but then became unhappy with him so she had changed it to her last name. It was so much better to use numbers.

We used our Vitek instrument to identify the org. The Vitek panels had the micro wells of chemicals which were then read after an incubation period and the computer decided from the various reactions the identity of the organism. There were separate panels for gram negative orgs, gram positive orgs and yeast. For bacteria, we also set up sensitivity panels with various antibiotics. If there was growth in the well, that meant the org was resistant to that particular antibiotic. If there was no growth, that antibiotic could be used against the infection. These reports went to the doctor with each antibiotic on the sensitivity report marked as sensitive, resistant or intermediate. Evening shift usually sent out the reports and there were hundreds of them every day. Along with workups, the blood culture tech was also loading the machines with new blood cultures as they came in. To top it off, at some time in the past, it had been decided that the blood culture bench would answer the phone which rang way too often. When I had my first surgery for breast cancer, years after my retirement, one of the nurses caring for me told me that I sounded familiar. I told her that I had worked in micro and she immediately remembered, "Oh, I've talked to you often. You always answered, 'Microbiology, Jo speaking.'"

We worked every other weekend in micro. In the main lab, it is often possible for techs to cover only every third weekend because the doctors do not regularly come in on the weekend so there are fewer orders but, in micro, what we set up on Friday had to "read," meaning the plates examined, and the panels set up the next day so Saturday was a busy day with fewer techs than usual.

The urine bench has the largest number of cultures. It is just too easy for the bladder to become infected, especially in patients who have indwelling catheters. I got the record number of plates when I worked that bench. There were eighteen plates (six sets of plates) in one of our metal cans and one morning I had thirty-seven cans. That record has since been far surpassed.

We were expected to examine all those plates in an eight hour shift, though the ones that had been set up later the evening before were not reported out until they had sufficient time to grow. With practice, the tech could open the plates, decide whether the bacteria was gram negative or positive according to which plates it grew on and the appearance of the colonies. There were also spot tests such as indole and oxidase for gram negative orgs or the catalase test to differentiate between staph and strep. If the plates grew a mix of common skin organisms, we suspected it was a contaminated sample, rather than a true infection. This could make the urine bench the most frustrating bench because we did not always get clean catch specimens. Urine in the bladder itself should be sterile but there are bacteria in the genital area that can contaminate the sample or, worse yet, some nursing staff just drained urine from the Foley bag which had been sitting for hours at room temperature with multiple bacteria growing in it instead of getting the sample aseptically directly from the Foley tube as they were supposed to do.

Most doctors would order a urinalysis with culture if indicated. This was a good idea when the urine was really infected as it allowed an immediate culture rather than waiting for the doctor to see the report and then order the culture later. However, if it was a contaminated sample, it could mean a messy and unnecessary culture. This kind of sloppy collection creates high cost in culturing urines that don't need it and possibly treating a patient who does not really have an infection.

In our lab, we had a bench dedicated to respiratory and stool specimens. Any sputum or throat culture should have growth as there is normal flora in the mouth and throat. If there was no growth from a sputum or throat, that was a red flag that the patient had been given too many antibiotics. Lack of normal flora left a breeding ground for pathogens. It took practice to be able to pick out the abnormal flora from all the rest but it was important as the doctor depended on us to find the organism causing pneumonia or perhaps strep throat.

Stools were challenging for me at first as the bad org can hide in normal flora in a stool. Salmonella is one of the pathogens we look for and it is one of the reportable diseases. There was a list of diseases that we were expected to subculture (streak a colony from an original plate to a new plate or slant and send the new culture with accompanying paperwork to the health department). The health department would then track down the source of the organism. I once had a positive salmonella culture from an infant. We duly sent a subbed culture plate to the health department and they ascertained that the parents of the baby kept pet snakes. Salmonella is normal flora in birds and snakes and they had apparently not been careful enough about washing their hands between caring for the snakes and then their baby.

There are multiple pathogens associated with stool cultures. In addition to salmonella or shigella which can be picked up on a regular culture, it was important to make sure that there was adequate growth of normal flora. We reported scant growth if the patient had been treated with something that suppressed the normal flora of the gut. Adequate nutrition is impossible without the help of our microbiota which actually do the absorption of nutrients. Some organisms, such as pseudomonas, could overgrow if normal flora was suppressed.

In addition, we set up special plates to recover *Vibrio vulnificus*. That is an organism found in seawater and it can contaminate oysters and possibly clams but raw oysters are the main culprit. Vibrio is found fairly often in Florida because of consumption of oysters that might be collected in areas of contaminated seawater. V. vulnifucus can also be contracted if you get contaminated seawater in an open wound.

Another pathogen was Campylobacter jejuni. This org required incubation of plates at a higher temperature. We had incubators set at the different temps required for specific organisms.

If it was ordered, we tested for Clostridium difficile, commonly abbreviated C. diff. This anaerobic organism was detected via a serological test at the time. It is a real problem in patients being treated with antibiotics and results in a nasty condition called pseudomembranous colitis. The diarrhea includes what appears to be tissue being sloughed off the intestine and can be fatal if not treated. Unfortunately, it is all too common in nursing homes and intensive care units where heavy duty antibiotics have been used.

Though E. coli is normal flora in the stool, there is a pathogenic form, E.coli O157:57, which causes a hemorrhagic diarrhea that can lead to damage of the blood vessels and even to kidney failure (Mayo Clinic, 2021). That is the organism that was in the news in 1993 when it was found in Jack in the Box hamburgers. This nasty bug made 700 people sick, with 171 hospitalizations and four deaths (News, 2017). We did find that organism on rare occasions.

One of the differences I found in working micro was the number of times I washed my hands. In the main lab, we usually only washed our hands when we took off our gloves, whether that was because we had specimen on them or because we were taking a meal break. In micro we were not encouraged to wear gloves when opening plates because the gloves had a tendency to stick to the plates and could carry bacteria from one plate to another. Instead, we washed our hands very often. The hospital supplied an antibacterial soap for our use but three of us, including me, developed an allergy to that soap. Our supervisor said it was required that techs use the antibacterial soap but we pointed out that using it resulted in broken skin, not a good thing when working with bacteria. We finally bought our own Softsoap and kept it under the sink.

Any time we had a wound on our hands, we were careful to keep it bandaged. One tech got MRSA in her finger and it was difficult to treat. I believe, of all the laboratory departments, working in micro carried the most risk of being infected with something we handled. We used needles to transfer blood from the blood culture bottles to the plates and one tech did get a needle stick when transferring. Though we set up everything but urines under a hood with filters and a laminar flow of air that was supposed to keep the aerosols contained, at times I could still smell the stools or specimens with gross infection when they were being set up so I know we were breathing it.

Night shift performed the ova and parasite exams. We do not see hookworm or roundworm in this country often anymore but pinworms are still around. Indeed, I once stained a small amount of a stool from a nursing home patient with methylene blue. The purpose was to look for white cells which would indicate inflammation in the gut. Imagine my surprise, when I looked down the barrels of the microscope and saw tiny worms crawling across the microscope field. The other techs laughed at me because I let out a yip when I saw the unexpected movement. I called the nursing home right away with the discovery, as pinworms are quite contagious.

A stool pathogen that is of particular concern to municipalities is cryptosporidium. Crypto is especially dangerous because it is not killed by ordinary chlorination of drinking water so it can be a real problem if it gets into the water supply. We tested with serological kits but the cysts can be detected with acid fast stains such as those used for TB.

I never worked the wound bench at this lab though I did work with wounds in other hospitals. Wound cultures are particularly challenging and only the most experienced micro techs worked that bench. Wound cultures are always set up both aerobically and anaerobically. It took experience to recognize the different colonies on a plate. Pathogens were often mixed with normal skin flora. The wound bench tech had to compare the aerobic with the anaerobic plate to tell if there was an org growing on the anaerobic plate that was not present aerobically. Usually, isolation required him or her to subculture each different looking colony both aerobically and anaerobically to differentiate the orgs. Isolation always had to be done before a panel could be set up. Only pure cultures would give a usable result.

I use the pronouns him or her because we did have male techs. They were fewer in number but they were all good techs and times had changed. When I trained and for many years after, almost all techs were female and all supervisors were male. Male techs made more than female techs then, ostensibly because they had families to support. That was the reasoning given. Of course, many female techs were supporting families, too, but that wasn't considered the norm so was ignored. I don't think there is pay discrepancy anymore between the sexes and many supervisors are female. My daughter and her 40-something friends find it hard to believe that women did not always have the opportunities they have now. They don't understand the purpose of the women's movement. "What was that all about, anyway?" they ask. They don't realize that it was precisely that movement that allows them their opportunities.

Female techs had to evolve, too. When the lab first became mechanized, many women would step back and expect the men to do repairs. I never thought this was fair. If we wanted to be paid equally, we had to learn to use tools. Some women also expected the male techs to do any heavy lifting. They would ask the men to lift the heavy boxes of saline we used for the hematology analyzers. The men never complained when asked but I learned to do it myself in two stages. I would lift it to a chair, then from the chair to the counter. Male techs would even be called for orderly duty elsewhere in the hospital. Bob tells me of an incident in his early years of working in the lab when a request came over the intercom for able-bodied male employees to assist in physical therapy. It turned out that a 400-pound patient had been lowered into a tub and they couldn't get her out. Bob went down and assisted in the effort though I am sure that was not in his job description.

PCR had come to the clinical lab. The hospital had hired an Italian dynamo with a doctorate to be in charge of this new technology. She was terrific. She began by holding classes in genetics. I had taken genetics more recently than many of the techs since I got my degree later in life but a refresher was needed so we would understand what we were doing. Polymerase chain reaction works by multiplying segments of a particular DNA fragment many times until there are enough of the fragments to be detected. The process was developed by Kary B. Mullis, an American biochemist who was born on a farm, like me, this one in rural North Carolina. He grew up wondering about the natural world around him and went on to win the Nobel prize in chemistry in 1993 for his work in developing PCR (editors, n.d.).

We started using PCR to detect MRSA (methicillin resistant staph aureus) DNA. The process we were previously using took too long to identify this pathogen since the doctor wanted to put any patient with MRSA in isolation as soon as possible to prevent spread. The drug needed to kill MRSA is expensive and has side effects. Resistance to it when overused is also to be avoided so hospitals do everything they can to keep it in check. We had been setting up a culture, letting it grow, then using appearance and catalase to identify staph, then setting up an ID panel to tell if it was S. aureus and setting up a sensitivity panel to see if it was resistant to methicillin. In all, that took at least two days. Two days while no special precautions were being taken to isolate the patient and the patient probably wasn't being treated with the heavy duty antibiotic needed to kill this tough org.

With the PCR method, a nasal swab was done on an incoming patient since MRSA colonizes the nasal passage creating a reservoir that could lead to MRSA in a wound or, worse yet, spread to another patient. Using this method, we could tell the doctor if it was MRSA in about two hours. There were no analyzers at that time to run the test. We used micro centrifuge tubes and multiple careful steps to get a result of positive or negative. The process had to be done in a room set aside for the purpose since we could not risk contamination with organisms in main micro. Today, PCR is used far more frequently for multiple pathogens using different primers and has been a godsend for diagnosis in the lab and for genetic testing. Analyzers have made the process much simpler but I'm glad I got in on the ground floor because I feel I had a better appreciation of the science.

Oh, and in addition to teaching us genetics and guiding all of us in this new technology, our mentor taught us how to make tiramisu and pesto.

The only department where I never worked was mycology. We set up yeasts in main micro but only the very experienced techs worked with fungi. Fungus cultures were set up on special agar, Sabouraud, often with antibiotics added to retard bacterial growth so the mold could be isolated. Yeasts are unicellular organisms that bud to form new growth but molds are multicellular and their filamentous structures must be studied both macro- and microscopically to identify the species. One tech, Debbie, had worked in Washington, D.C. She took a course in mycology at NIH (National Institutes of health) and had seen the infections that people could contract overseas. It took real skill to recognize the different molds on a plate and under a scope. Mycology has become more important since the advent of AIDS. Those patients had no resistance to ordinary molds such as those found in soil and molds even showed up in blood cultures.

The TB room was a separate negative pressure room, meaning no air went out of it when the door was opened. Special machines similar to the blood culture machines agitated the TB cultures and there was an alarm if one was positive. One tech was assigned to this room. We did direct smears on all specimens but a positive was far more likely after incubation in a growth medium. Positive specimens were stained and the ID determined. Sensitivities had to be sent out to National Jewish Laboratories as we did not then have the technology to do them inhouse.

Next I learned virology. It was a whole new world and I was glad for the opportunity to learn it because a tech can get a little tired of looking at the same common pathogens day after day. For virology, the patient specimen could be from a nasal swab if looking for a respiratory virus, from a lesion if looking for herpes or from body fluid such as spinal fluid. We could detect cytomegalovirus (cmv), herpes, adenovirus, influenzas A and B, respiratory syncytial virus (RSV)and parainfluenza. A growth medium was inoculated with the specimen and it was allowed to grow in the medium. We then used what were called shell vials. In the bottom of each flat-bottomed vial was a membrane of media which would grow the virus in question.

Viruses only grow in living tissue and different viruses required different tissue. Common types of cell lines in use were monkey kidney cells, embryonic cells and epithelial cells. Doctors could order a specific virus culture or they could order a panel. Three vials were set up for each virus type ordered on one patient. We wanted to catch the virus growth as soon as possible but, with the exception of herpes, most times it took more than one day for the virus to grow enough to be detected. By having three, we could examine one shell vial each day for three days. For the enteric viruses, the ones that often cause diarrhea in kids, we started staining on the third day and gave them five days.

It was a delicate procedure. First the inoculated culture was centrifuged after incubation and the sediment "button" from the bottom transferred to the proper shell vial which had a minimum amount of growth medium in it to keep moisture present. The vial was centrifuged to force the virus onto the membrane at the bottom. Then the vial was incubated. Herpes could be detected in the shortest time, 18–24 hours via a technology called ELVIS. Herpes I is the virus that causes cold sores, but it can cause genital herpes. Herpes II causes genital herpes and it is one of the most common sexually transmitted diseases. We detected any virus after growth by carefully peeling off the membrane from the bottom of the vial and putting it on a slide, then introducing an antibody specific to the virus in question.

Virology had its own room and its own hood to use for this process. The membrane was then stained with a fluorescent stain, and examined under a fluorescent microscope. Of course, we could not see the actual virus as they are much too small but we saw the cytopathic effect when the dye-tagged antibody met the antigen of the virus. Bright green patches would glow under the scope and you knew you had a positive result. RSV was particularly easy to detect because the cells run together (that's why they call it syncytial) and a large area will glow.

The virus bench usually did not take all day so we used the afternoons to put away media. It came in by the truckload in fairly large boxes and similar kinds of plates had to be stored together. Media also had to be rotated so the oldest was used first. We had a walk-in cooler but it was always a struggle to get everything in the cooler in the proper order. ID and sensi panels for the Vitek also had to be stocked and new lot numbers recorded so QC could be done before a new lot was used.

A new tech learns very early to put things away in their proper place so that other techs can find what they need in a hurry. Not everyone adhered to this principle. At other labs, I have reached into a drawer for a new probe when one bent and come up with another one that was also bent and had not been thrown away. When a patient's life may be at stake, you don't want to have to search for a part, timer or pipettes because someone else did not put it back where it belonged.

The daily running of micro was done by a few senior techs. They did the scheduling since we all rotated through several benches making sure plenty of people were cross trained. There was never any reason for anyone to say, "Oh, we can't do that test. So and so is off today." That won't fly in the clinical lab. The senior techs monitored the QC and there was a lot of it. We set up panels on known purchased organisms to prove our biochemistry panels and sensitivity panels were accurate. Sometimes, we needed to do manual sensitivities, called E tests, which were occasionally necessary if the machine failed us or for organisms that did not have panels. We used an agar specifically for sensitivity and the E test strips were imbedded with various antibiotics. Controls had to be done to prove the efficacy of our agar and strips. Controls were run on the kit tests. There were positive and negative control slides for gram stains. Records had to be kept on all of this and that fell to the senior techs.

When we had inspections, whether for JCAHO or CAP, it was the senior techs who took the inspector through the lab, opened the procedure manuals for the inspector, showed them the licensure for all of those working in micro and took responsibility for correcting any discrepancy. They did all this and they manned their own bench as well almost every day. These senior techs were my lifeline. They were all great but I remember one, in particular, who showed so much patience when I was learning to read viral fluorescent stains. I was so afraid that I would miss a positive, that I dragged her away from her own work multiple times to go look through the fluorescent microscope in another room until I felt confident in reporting without her help. Oh, and she made wonderful Indian food to share with us.

There were CAP surveys to be done in micro. These were unknown samples that we plated or ran via kits to prove our methods were adequate. CAP also sent pictures of bioterrorism agents that we were supposed to watch for. It reminded us that we could be setting up bacillus anthracis (anthrax), yersinia pestis (plague) or brucella, all highly contagious organisms we could be setting up and working with on open plates before we could identify them.

Some months before I retired, we were told that the entire department of microbiology would be relocating to a sister hospital in another city. Management felt that it would save money to consolidate machines and techs in one facility. Of course, we did not like it. Some of those techs had worked in micro for thirty years and their reward was to have to drive to another facility every morning. The move finally happened after I had retired. I was told that it was crowded in the new facility and techs in the existing lab had their own way of doing things so compromises had to be worked out. No one was happy about it as the techs at the new lab lost their space when our machines and people had to be accommodated. The doctors were not happy, either, when their specimens had to be driven a distance before they could be plated and allowed to grow but once again, medicine is a business and I saw the same thing happen in other micro labs. Of course, in time, new ways of doing things were worked out and results became more timely.

I retired at the age of 69 in 2014. I had taken a PRN (as needed) position when I turned 62 and started drawing social security. In retrospect, this was a mistake because the law at that time only allowed me to make the $15,000/yr. before sacrificing benefits. I should have waited until full retirement age so that my benefit would have been higher. Because I went on working and paying into the system, my benefit did increase but perhaps not to the amount it would have been had I waited. I don't believe there should be a limit on the amount social security beneficiaries make because people need to go on working to supplement and because skilled workers are still needed. At 66, full retirement age for me, I was no longer limited as to what I could make so I started working a lot of hours but without any employee benefits. PRN pay is higher but the position does not qualify for vacation or sick time. I often worked six days a week as a PRN.

The night that I decided to retire, I was still working at a second job, also PRN, in the main lab of a sister hospital. One evening, I had gone into the break room to eat my dinner and picked up a newspaper. While perusing the obituaries, I was stunned to see that one of my teachers in junior college, himself a birder, had died. I was stunned. He was no older than I was. It suddenly dawned on me that I was getting up in years. Merle had long ago retired but we couldn't do much traveling because of my schedule. I worried that I would not have enough in savings to last for my lifetime but I also realized that I might never feel that I had enough. I went to the computer and emailed my supervisors in both hospitals that I was retiring in one month.

The other techs gave me a great party when I left. I was touched that they remembered that my favorite cake was lemon and that I liked flowers. There was a lovely bouquet. My husband and I were planning a trip to Australia and the break room was decorated with pictures of Sydney and Australian wildlife. It was a bittersweet day.

Interview with a Molecular Tech (2023), Post-Covid

Please tell us your name, shift and duties.

My name is Carolyn Dowell. I work second shift in a molecular lab. I have worked in the clinical lab for 37 yrs.

What do you feel is the biggest challenge in your job?

I find that I have to work independently. Sometimes I am alone in the lab on my shift. There is no one to ask so I have to use my best judgment if there is a decision to be made. I can text my manager or director but they are not always immediately available. This can be stressful since what we do is important to the patient.

Is your job different since Covid? How did it affect you?

It's better now but it was terrible during Covid. I was working at a hospital during that period. Covid tests took priority over other tests. The other tests had to wait. We didn't like feeling that we were getting behind on the other testing. And there was the setting up before we could even get the sample on the instrument. We had to open the swabs under the hood while wearing our regular fluid impermeable lab coat, gloves, mask and an additional face shield. We all felt hot in this attire. Then we had to be very careful when transferring the processed samples to the instrument. I had to ask everyone to clear the room and I shut the doors so that any spill would be contained. Only after the transfer of the samples to the instrument was complete could we open the doors.

In molecular, where I later started working, we had to get FDA permission to run two specimens mixed together in the interest of time and to conserve our reagents. If the combined sample was negative, we knew both patients were negative. If the combined sample was positive, each patient had to be set up individually and run again. Using this technique, we could run 188 samples per run. I ran four of these double runs in one evening, that's 752 Covid tests by myself.

How do you feel that working in the lab affected your personal life?

I was able to stay home with my children when they were small but, when they got older, there were times when I needed to be in two places at once. My daughter called me at work one day to say that she had broken a glass while washing dishes. She didn't know whether she would need stitches. I had to leave work and found that she did need stitches. My husband did not do much to help out but I found ways to take care of the kids while still working. One strategy was to buy ramen noodles. The kids liked them and the snack kept them from being too hungry before I could get home and cook dinner. Both of my parents worked fulltime but sometimes I could use them for childcare on weekends.

Do you feel that you are recognized as part of the healthcare team?

It's better since Covid. It took Covid to make the team realize the lab existed. During the epidemic, nurses would have to bring the samples from the floors to the lab as they were not allowed to use the tube system to send them. They could see how many tests we were running. Also, lab personnel had to go to the ER for any Covid specimens being taken there. That took techs away from the bench in order to collect those specimens.

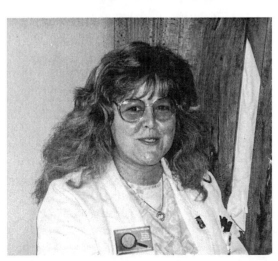

Carolyn Dowell, MT

Do you feel satisfaction in your work? Are you glad you went into the field?

I really loved my work for most of my

career but Covid squelched my passion. Maybe it was age but it exhausted me.

Would you recommend that young people go into this line of work?

I'm not sure that I could encourage a young person to go into lab work. We have people with four-year degrees in the sciences that come to work as LMAs (lab assistants). These are starter positions that don't pay as much. It gives them a taste of what lab work is but they have to continue to go to school and take an additional 15–16 months of training before they can take the test to be techs. I advise them not to do that unless they really love the work. Many do not go on but, fortunately, some continue. There is a real shortage of techs now. Recruiters ask for experience but the experienced techs are retiring and new techs don't have experience yet. Labs are offering bonuses if a tech will work for two years but I have seen some who put in the two years, get the experience, then go to another lab that is offering another bonus. I don't know who is going to be doing this work in the future.

TWELVE

The Lab of Today
and Tomorrow

Even before I retired, new organisms had become problems. In hematology, techs had to examine white blood cells for the inclusions of ehrlichiosis and anaplasmosis, tickborne diseases caused by the bite of the Lone Star tick in the case of ehrlichiosis and of the deer tick in anaplasmosis (Petri, 2022). Now immunofluorescence has taken over the job of finding these infections.

There are now instruments to better streamline care in hematology. With the instrument currently in use at my former place of employment, a blood sample is aspirated and the machine determines all the parameters of a CBC. If they are all normal, the report goes out without any further attention from a tech. If any abnormality is detected, the machine makes a slide, stains the slide, and, using a new methodology called CellaVision, looks at the cells with an indwelling microscope and flashes the cells it has seen onto a computer screen. The tech can immediately identify the abnormality by looking at the screen and the need for a manual differential is eliminated.

CellaVision has the advantage of allowing multiple people to view the same cells on the screen at the same time and the screen can be pulled up at any computer station in the lab so that, if a night shift tech is running more than one bench, he does not need to go to the hema station to review the slide, saving many steps. Many manual diffs are still done, however, because CellaVision cannot be totally trusted to identify very abnormal cells. Not yet, anyway. My guide estimates that manual differentials have been reduced by at least 85 percent. You will remember that it used to keep one tech busy all shift doing diffs. Cerebrospinal fluid counts can be done on the instrument. It will tell the tech the number of white cells and red cells and differentiate the white cells by type. Joint fluids are usually too viscous and are done manually.

In urinalysis, the Velocity instrument reads the chemical reactions in urines while the Iris instrument has mostly eliminated the microscopic examination of urine sediment. This instrument, too, projects cells onto a screen for techs to identify. The company claims that it reduces tech time by 78 percent (writers, 2021). Of course, techs still need to look under the scope if there is an indication of a problem.

In chemistry, there is a high sensitivity troponin. I've read that biomarkers for celiac disease and multiple sclerosis have been developed and there is a test for serum amyloid which is said to be a better marker for inflammation than the tests we have been doing.

I toured the chemistry department at the same hospital and was very impressed with their robotic line which brings tubes directly to the instrument from processing. The Accelerator A3600 by Abbott is truly self-contained. If a tube that needs centrifugation has not been spun, the machine can sense this and sends the tube to an indwelling centrifuge. The machine uncaps the tubes, reducing the aerosols that were generated when techs opened vacuum tubes themselves. Using this system, the ordered test is automatically sent to the proper instrument, run on it and, if normal, the results go out without further tech attention. The machine can even do dilutions and, for absolute security of sample identity, the machine takes a picture of the tube with its barcode so there can be no doubt as to what tube was tested.

If a TSH, the initial test for thyroid function, is run and found to be abnormal, it institutes a thyroid cascade so that a T4, Free T4 and T3 can be automatically done, saving time and getting a diagnosis for the patient sooner. Specimens are stored on the instrument at the appropriate temperature. If an additional test is ordered on an existing specimen, the machine finds the specimen and runs it with no human involvement. The machine has a sealing function where it heats a small piece of foil and seals the tubes after they have been run. If the tube is needed again, there is a separate station for unsealing them. When the specimen has been stored for the maximum amount of time that integrity can be assured, the machine even dumps the expired tubes into a biohazard container.

BNPs have become a standard test now. B-type natriuretic peptide is an indicator of heart function. If the heart has to pump too hard, the BNP rises. The Architect instrument made by Abbott runs cyclosporine.

Cyclosporine is used to combat rejection of organ transplants but also to treat autoimmune diseases as it reduces immune response. The Architect is also capable of running tests for syphilis which is said to have increased in incidence by 66.7 percent (Healthcare, 2017).

In coagulation, the methodology is similar to what was in use when I was working, that is a photo optical method of detecting clot formation. However, the instrument now can sense if the volume is too low in the tube, a very important factor in coag since the ratio of anti-coagulant to sample is crucial. The machine can also detect lipemia and hemolysis.

This new automation has reduced the need for techs. My guide told me that they now have six techs running hema, coag and chem where they used to need nine on day shift. Night shift runs with four techs. However, techs have become increasingly hard to find. Many hospitals are still using what are called traveling techs such as Nancy mentioned in her interview. These are techs who work through an agency that sends techs where laboratories need them. They are considerably more expensive than regularly employed techs but the hospital has had no choice. Probably in response to the demand, my former hospital has begun offering flexible scheduling. If a tech wishes, he or she can work 12-hour days, an option that was never available where I worked.

In Blood Bank, electronic crossmatches have been being done for years. Our computer system was programmed to prevent any ABO incompatible blood from going out to the patient. All recipient samples are screened for antibodies and their history is researched for previous antibodies. All donor units are rechecked for group and type. If there is no antibody in the recipient, the two are electronically matched and a unit of their group and type is chosen. If the two are compatible, the blood is issued with tech and nurse still reviewing and checking before dispensing. We were all a little apprehensive when this system came about but it has proven to be safe and it has cut the time it takes to get the blood to where it needs to go.

In addition, blood banks now use apheresis to separate blood components. Blood can be separated into packed red blood cells; plasma, platelet concentrates, leukocyte (white blood cell) concentrates and cryoprecipitate. This can be done while the donor is still in the chair with the desired component separated from the whole blood and the rest of the blood returned to the donor. In this way, more blood can be filtered for the desired component without taking too much blood volume from the donor.

Platelet concentrates are used for people with platelet deficiency or for platelet immunization problems. Cryoprecipitate is needed for people with clotting problems and leukocyte concentrations are used for people with chronic low white blood cell conditions. Component concentrates are often irradiated with gamma radiation to avoid reactions to the antigens that they contain. This step avoids immunizing the recipient to foreign antigens and making it possible for that individual to continue to receive concentrated components. Sometimes the white blood cells are separated from the blood components to avoid immunization to the HLA (human leukocyte antigens) that white blood cells contain (Basu, 2014). Fresh frozen plasma is always kept on hand because it can be given quickly and it contains clotting properties.

Blood bank techs are in demand and our local blood supply company offers opportunities for paid training in exchange for agreeing to work in the field for them for a specified period of time.

I don't know of any doctor's office that does not receive their lab results directly to their laptop computers usually overnight and most patients can see their results at home on their patient portal via the internet. No more waiting for the courier to bring reports and no more need for bulky printed patient files. Every doctor in the system has access to the patient records written on that patient by other doctors in the same system so there is less chance of two doctors prescribing similar or the same drugs and thus overdosing the patient.

For some time now, testing has been moving to the patient bedside. It began with the little Accuchek blood sugar testing machines. Now, there are watches that detect the patient's blood sugar level through the skin, noninvasively. We refer to bedside testing as point of care testing or POCT. Companies such as Abbott make handheld instruments with cartridges that can run coagulation tests, electrolytes, troponin and CK-MB, hematocrit or creatinine at the bedside. They claim most tests take about two minutes and the result can be transmitted to the laboratory computer wirelessly. I can see how this technology at the bedside would be great for a dialysis patient to get his creatinine level immediately before his treatment or for an initial diagnosis of a heart attack or a bleed in an emergency setting but this technology is expensive and will probably never replace the clinical lab where so many samples can be run in batches at less cost.

Elaine, who was in charge of point of care testing during her career, says, "It was the collaboration of the laboratory department and the nursing department that brought point of care testing to the forefront. The laboratory initiated the testing devices, coordinated the training of the nurses and provided the quality control of the reagents to satisfy regulatory guidelines. These testing panels greatly reduced the turn-around time for glucose monitoring, electrolyte panels, cardiac markers, pregnancy tests, urinalysis and strep screens to name a few. While speed and efficiency is vital, it is important to keep in mind that POCT was designed to screen for critical results to be confirmed later in the central lab."

So the lab is still intimately involved in bedside testing. Nurses are in short supply and adding POCT to their other duties without the lab's assistance in maintaining quality control and procedure would not make the nursing profession any more attractive.

There are now rapid tests for identifying TB. One uses PCR and is a wonderful method but I don't see how it could be used at missions in the developing world which might not even have electricity or, like mine, only the electricity that could be generated by a two foot by one foot solar panel. The other is a test for the TB antigen. The NIH tested one of these rapid tests on sputum and pleural fluid. The sensitivity was not great. Slightly more than half of the patients who had positive results using PCR also showed positive with the rapid test by BioMed labs, India. However, the sensitivity was much better if there was a heavy bacterial load (Grover, 2011). It seems to me that the test might be of use in a mission such as mine because the bacterial load was usually high and it would not require costly machinery or even much technical expertise

In the micro lab, a technology called Maldi-Tof is being used to identify bacteria. MALDI-TOF is the short form for matrix assisted laser desorption/ionization time of flight. It uses laser technology to identify organisms via analytical mass spectrometry and compares the results to known profiles of various organisms. It is cheaper than using the ID panels we used in Vitek and a lot of samples can be imbedded in the tiny wells of the sample plates used on the machine. Research is being done on expanding the use of MALDI to TB and fungi (Savelieff, 2018).

Also in micro, they now use a machine called the Verigene system. It uses what they call NanoGrid technology. The machine can extract nucleic acids and amplify them via PCR. It can identify the pathogen in a positive blood culture directly, no culture required, and also give the genes that organism carries for resistance to the important antibiotics. Their claim is to ID three staphs, three streps, enterococcus, micrococcus and listeria. It can ID nine gram negative orgs, the most important ones, and looks for resistance to six antibiotics. And this instrument does all this in two and a half hours! Compare this to the five days we gave any blood culture to turn positive, the time it took to grow the org on a culture plate, at least one full day, then the time it took to run the ID panel and sensitivities. What a boon to doctors and patients is the ability to report the resistance genes that necessitate patient sequestration and particular care in handling. Antibiotic resistance is escalating and information like this is what is needed to limit the nastiest pathogens that hospitals so dread and strive to contain.

Even these machines are not the latest technology. My source tells me that micro staff found themselves doing correlations on three new instruments at the same time during her employment. Imagine the amount of sample running of hundreds of specimens that I described earlier when doing validation studies times three. One new instrument is called the Bruker which is a similar technology to the MALDI-TOF but techs and management will decide which is the best for their purposes and for the patients after the correlations have been completed.

The Varigene website advertises that they also have technology for identifying respiratory pathogens but this lab uses another technology by Biofire. This instrument can identify all of the respiratory pathogens, stool pathogens, yeasts, viruses and parasites, directly from the sample, no culture, in less than an hour! In addition, Biofire also gives the resistance genes we mentioned before.

I was privileged to see the new technology for myself on a visit to the microbiology facility that serves our area. I watched the WASP (walk away specimen processor) robotic system that sets up the cultures. I saw it unscrew the top from the sample tube, streak the plate, wash itself and move on to the next. That machine makes the repetitive job of setting up cultures obsolete and frees lab personnel to take on other work.

A former coworker who is now in administration, took me through the micro section and told me about a spot test for methicillin resistance called PBP2 done in minutes on the bench, even faster than PCR.

She also told me about the QuantiFERON Gold test which has replaced skin tests to detect the antibody to TB in staff and all techs are now screened this way every year unless they have already tested positive for the antibody in the past. In that case, they would still need chest X-rays to rule out active disease. TB is still cultured if ordered on patients and they do get positives for M. tuberculosis as well as M. avium and M. abscessus.

Perhaps the most impressive change in the clinical lab has come about with the increased use of molecular studies. The head of esoteric took me through this building with the departments FISH, cytogenetics, flow cytometry, molecular studies and special chemistry.

I was most impressed with the FISH technology. FISH is the acronym for fluorescent in situ hybridization. I watched as the tech called up a tissue sample from a breast cancer patient. The tissue had been stained with a fluorescent probe to look for defects or changes in specific genes. The computer "maps" the genes, allowing the doctor to know, for one thing, whether the tumor is HER positive or negative and tailoring the treatment to suit. This is just one example of this amazing technology. But, since about one in eight American women will get breast cancer (CDC, Bring Your Brave, 2021) and, as a breast cancer survivor myself, this methodology is especially meaningful.

Molecular oncology has allowed doctors to use targeted therapy for patients by finding out exactly which biomarkers are on their specific tumor. Some drugs are known to work better for specific biomarkers so cancer treatment does not have to be the shotgun approach that used to be the only option. Also, molecular technology can be used for the formulation of antibodies to a specific cancer. Those antibodies would attack the cancer cells at the cellular level.

Flow cytometry is being done in the esoteric lab. That means faster results on the CD4 counts needed by HIV patients. This flow cytometry also detects abnormal cells in blood and bone marrow, helping to diagnose the various leukemias. For instance, it can pinpoint the BCR/ABL gene specific to chronic myelogenous leukemia. This technology works in tandem with pathologists and physicians who have the clinical picture.

PCR technology is used to identify acid fast bacilli such as TB and it also gives information about resistance to the most important antibiotics for those organisms.

DiaSorin technology allows the lab to run extracted specimens for Herpes I and II as well as Varicella zoster which is the virus that causes chicken pox and shingles. It can run spinal fluids for the viruses directly. Their website advertises kits for monkey pox. I was pleased to see that this instrument can identify bacteria that could be used for bio-terrorism. The website for DiaSorin advertises that they have probes for the bacteria that cause anthrax, botulism, valley fever and plague (Bannister, 2022). There is so much less risk using molecular methods than there is to grow these organisms out on plates with all the attendant exposure before the tech can know that she is dealing with a lethal bug.

The Cobas 6800 can run entire viral panels in three hours along with the sexually transmitted diseases. It identifies HIV, hepatitis B and C, cytomegalovirus, chlamydia, gonorrhea, human papilloma virus, trichomonas vaginalis and, of course, Covid. So much faster and more sensitive than the old shell vials.

The BD MAX instrument identifies via PCR technology an entire array of stool pathogens, bacterial and viral, including giardia and cryptosporidium in one go and also does panels on spinal fluid for meningitis. All this info can be released in three hours.

Immunoelectrophoresis has been mechanized to detect allergies as well as autoimmune disease. This methodology is being used to test for fecal occult blood instead of the card tests we used to do. The method is more likely to detect colon cancer at an earlier stage.

I was somewhat surprised to see so many regular cultures being done in micro with all the new methods available in molecular but it was explained that doctors still order cultures. It takes time for doctors to learn about and feel comfortable with molecular methods and it is also possible that the new methods are more costly. But I believe the time will come when culturing may be a thing of the past.

The interactive computer system has blossomed to include easier ways to communicate across the many hospitals and outpatient centers in the system. The supervisor showed me how she can see a gram stain which some tech in a distant facility needs help identifying in real time on her own screen in her office. She has a system that detects corrections made in Cerner so she can pinpoint if tech training is needed at another or at her own facility. If necessary, she can change the tech schedule on her phone which interfaces with the online scheduling system. Supervisors in the different facilities can come together in what they call huddles to discuss issues or new technology without leaving their desks. This lab, as well as other system labs, are accredited by CAP, the College of American Pathologists. Competencies are still required such as we used to do with CEUs but these educational modules are available in a system called MediaLab accessible at the techs' bench and the supervisor can call up a list of those who have done their competencies and those who have not.

Even the smaller hospitals in the system are running the GeneXpert and the Biofire Torch. The Biofire can run a panel so, if the Covid is negative, it can test the specimen further to detect RSV, flu, enterovirus or rhinovirus. Not having to do separate orders saves time and gives the doctor the info he needs to diagnose in one fell swoop.

There is no better example of the dedication exhibited by lab personnel than what happened during the Covid epidemic. Did you ever wonder who was running all those swabs taken everywhere on thousands of people? *Forbes* magazine reports that there were 997 million diagnostic tests done for Covid by laboratory professionals since the epidemic began (Stone, 2022). I have learned from former colleagues, some retired and some still working, about how it was during Covid and the situation has been discussed in the interviews in this book. The system for whom I worked had already bought a building to use for molecular studies as so many tests were now being done using PCR and related technology. After the micro department where I was employed had been moved to another hospital, it was decided that it would make more sense for all of the testing to be done in one place so all of micro moved again into the same building as molecular, now called the esoteric lab.

Many of those swabs for Covid went to this lab. Much credit should go to the techs who knocked themselves out during the Covid epidemic. Carolyn, working at the esoteric lab, says that their lab ran as many as 1100 Covid tests in just two shifts during the height of the epidemic and she has run over 700 by herself in one shift, sitting on the same lab stool and working with the samples under a hood for hours at a time, not only dressed in her normal lab coat but also wearing a fluid impermeable gown over the lab coat. In addition, she had to wear a mask and a face shield over the mask. It was hot and repetitive work but lab techs persevered throughout the epidemic. This esoteric lab was running that test on their very expensive Diasorin BD MAX and Cobas 6800 analyzers. The pressure was on and the phone calls never stopped while patients awaited their results. In addition, stat orders for Covid tests were done at every member hospital on other machines. These smaller hospitals were also swamped with Covid tests. But, when heroes were applauded during the epidemic, lab techs were never mentioned, though it was they who were handling the infectious samples and running them day and night for the duration. The lab was definitely on the front line during this emergency and it will be in the ones to come

I began in an era, not only pre computer, we didn't even have calculators! It was a forty year learning curve for me and for all those like me. Techs are becoming fewer in number, since so many of us are retiring and some laboratory training programs have closed. The molecular lab does not hire anyone without a four year degree. If the degree is in another science, Molecular trains them in the new methodology and they take additional courses so they can qualify for registry, making them eligible for Florida licensure. Hillsborough Community College works with area hospitals to train medical laboratory assistants, who are not licensed when they come to work but they can continue their academic courses and can obtain licensure after enough experience and training. Still, there are always openings. I counted 39 lab positions of various levels for one medical consortium today and I know other hospitals are also looking for techs and other personnel. *Forbes* reports that there was a shortage in 2022 of 20,000–25,000 techs in the U.S. (Stone, 2022).

There is good reason for this. I have said that I began my career making just over a dollar an hour. With forty years of experience and licensing in six specialties, I was finally making $28 an hour when I left the lab in 2014. If I worked fulltime but on a PRN basis (so with no benefits) I could rack up about $50,000 a year. I had chosen to work on a PRN basis after I qualified for medicare as I did not need the health insurance offered by the hospital. I also thought I would have more flexibility in my schedule as a PRN but I found it hard to refuse when other techs needed time off and there was no one else to cover for them. Some other techs, working fulltime as regular employees and with just as much experience, were not making as much as I was.

It was not until I started drawing Social Security that I realized how I had hurt myself by not trying out for supervisory positions that would have paid more. I paid into the Social Security system for 46 years but I drew less than $1000 a month when I began drawing the benefit at age 62. It is something to think about when you are working. The more you make, the more your benefit will be. Working women are not compensated as they should be. Non-working spouses are eligible for a spousal benefit that is half again of their husband's benefit. That is not half of his. He will receive the full amount he is due. She is eligible for an amount equal to one half of the amount he draws so that, together, they are drawing one and one half times the benefit he earned. This rule was made many years ago when few spouses worked. I'm sure it was fair at the time but now the rule allows the wealthiest of women, who never had to work, to receive a benefit while those who worked must sacrifice their spousal benefit as you are not allowed to draw both. I would get almost the same amount as the wife of a retiree, had I never worked, as I am getting for working and paying into social security for 46 years. And the non-working spouse did not have to pay for childcare from her wages.

The new term for a medical technologist is clinical laboratory scientist. This new term came into use because there were other workers in other medical disciplines also called medical technologists and the new title needed to include the word laboratory. Various websites differ in reporting salaries for clinical laboratory scientists today but the average is about $58,483. The pay has gone up, certainly, but the starting salary of a young man I know working in software sales is $85,000 a year. That is starting salary. He will be eligible for bonuses amounting to the same amount again. And he didn't have to suffer through calculus and physics!

As I've said before, we work incognito and we don't have a good lobby. Young people are often not aware of laboratory work as a career or, if they are, they might feel that it doesn't pay enough to compensate for the grueling training in the sciences, the hospital hours with attendant childcare problems and there is the fact that you may be exposed to transmissible disease though the new safety protocols make that far less likely.

Though lab work may not pay the best, there are rewards and they are many. I don't regret my choice of career. I loved the work and I know I did help patients. I kept my brain active and I was part of the medical arsenal even if unseen. I have noticed, too, that doctors have changed. My great aunt told me that when she trained as a nurse in the early twentieth century, nurses were expected to stand up when the doctor entered the room. Doctors were gods and, even when I began my career, they could be very autocratic. Suggestions from a lowly tech were not usually welcomed. Now, the younger doctors would call micro and ask advice on which antibiotic they should give and they were far more patient when we had to call them on the weekends. It seemed that they were finally seeing techs as part of the team.

There is more versatility in lab work now. Molecular offers a new field and I know techs who have staffed fertility clinics working with sperm and egg to help childless couples. There is work in government agencies such as the CDC and in industries such as food processing. Some techs get jobs with the instrument companies, either selling the technology or traveling around and training new users when they get the instrument.

Lab jobs are out there. I never had to look long for a job and there are even more positions open now. I made a living wage and I made wonderful friends, my fellow techs, for whom I have the greatest respect. I can quite honestly recommend that young people go into the field and my interviews show that other techs feel the same. I hope this book has helped to educate the public about the professional people behind those laboratory doors who first have to learn the science, then use all that ever-changing technology and keep it going 24/7.

In *Forbes* magazine, Dr. Rodney Rohde, professor of clinical lab science at Texas State University, said, "Lab testing is the single highest-volume medical activity affecting Americans.... Simply put, every time you enter a hospital or healthcare facility for care, your life is in the hands of a medical laboratory professional (Stone, 2022)."

You may not see us but we are there for you.

Bibliography

ARUP, L.O. (2022, October). *ARUP Consult.* "Sjogren Syndrome." https://arupconsult. com/content/sjogren-syndrome.

Bactec Newsletter. (2014, July). "Flourescent Technology in the BD." http://www.bmsd. com.my/files/editor_files/file/July-2014.pdf.

Bannister, C. (2022, March 11). *Luminex.* "Four Types of Pathogenic Bacteria Used in Bioterrorism." https://www.luminexcorp.com/blog/4-types-of-pathogenic-bacteria-used-in-bioterrorism/.

Barbara May Foundation. (2023). "Save the Mother, Save the World." https:// barbaramayfoundation.com/.

Basu, K. (2014, September-October 2014). *NIH Library of Medicine.* "Overview of Blood Components and Their Preparation." https://www.ncbi.nlm.nih.gov/pmc/articles/ PMC4260297/.

Buttner, J. (1992, October 30). *Eur J Clin Chem Clin Biochem.* "The Origin of Clinical Laboratories." Nat. Laboratory of Medicine, PubMed.gov. https://pubmed.ncbi.nlm. nih.gov/1493151/.

CDC. (1982, March 19). *MMWR.* "Historical Perspective Centennial on Koch's Discovery of the Tubercule Bacteria." https://www.cdc.gov/mmwr/preview/mmwrhtml/ 00000222.htm.

CDC. (2021, September 27). *Bring Your Brave.* "Breast Cancer in Young Women." https:// www.cdc.gov/cancer/breast/young_women/bringyourbrave/breast_cancer_young_ women/index.htm#:~:text=Breast%20cancer%20is%20the%20most,under%20the%20 age%20of%2045.

CDC. (2022, June 22). "Health Insurance Portability Act." https://www.cdc.gov/phlp/ publications/topic/hipaa.html.

CDC. (2022, October 18). "Fast Facts: GB Can Be Very Serious, Especially for Babies." https://www.cdc.gov/groupbstrep/about/fast-facts.html#:~:text=GBS%20disease%20 can%20be%20very,the%20bacteria%20late%20in%20pregnancy.

CDC. (2018, November 15). "*Strengthening Clinical Labs.*" https://www.cdc.gov/csels/ dls/strengthening-clinical-labs.html.

Collins, K. (2017, December 13). *Eureka.* "Thanks to the Power of Blue Blood." https:// www.criver.com/eureka/blue-blood.

Cross, A.R. (2023). *American Red Cross.* "FAQ'S." https://www.redcrossblood.org/ faq.html#:~:text=How%20long%20will%20it%20take,required%20between%20 whole%20blood%20donations.

Doctors Without Borders. (2022). "Our History." https://www.doctorswithoutborders. org/who-we-are/our-history.

editors. (n.d.). *The Nobel Prize.* "Kary B. Mullis Facts." https://www.nobelprize.org/ prizes/chemistry/1993/mullis/facts/.

Eldridge, L.M. (2022, September 13). *Verywell Health.* "An Overview of the Thymus Gland." https://www.verywellhealth.com/thymus-gland-overview-4582270.

Bibliography

Encyclopaedia Britannica. (2022, June 22). "Karl Landsteiner." https://www.britannica.com/biography/Karl-Landsteiner. Accessed November 21, 2022.

Fisher Science. (2017, February 10). *Abbot Architect Syphilis Testing.* "Syphilis on the Rise." https://www.fishersci.com/content/fishersci/en_US/healthcare-products/selection-guides/clinical-analyzers-instruments/fast-reliable-results-abbott-architect-assays/abbott-architect-syphilis-testing.html.

Food Safety News. (2017, December 27). "Jack in the Box E Coli Outbreak." https://www.foodsafetynews.com/2017/12/jack-in-the-box-e-coli-outbreak-25th-anniversary/.

Grover, L.S. (2011, July 21). *NIH.* "Detection of TB Antigen by Rapid Test." https://www.ncbi.nlm.nih.gov/pmc/articles/PMC4920755/.

Hassan, C. (2022, September 21). *CNN Health.* "Cancer Deaths Fall Steadily in the US with More Survivors Than Ever." https://www.cnn.com/2022/09/21/health/cancer-deaths-decline-research-report/index.html.

Hayes, E. (2020, February 24). *Lab Pulse.* "Surveys Shine Light on Stress, Burnout in Lab Professionals." https://www.labpulse.com/diagnostic-technologies/pathology-and-ai/pathology-histology/article/15298445/surveys-shine-light-on-stress-burnout-in-lab-professionals.

Hematology, W.M. (n.d.). *McGraw-Hill Medical.* "Laboratory Variables."

Hole, J.W. (1978). *Human Anatomy and Physiology.* Dubuque, Iowa: Wm. C. Brown Co.

Horsti, J. (2009, July 1). PubMed Central. "The Progress of Prothrombin Time Measurement." https://www.ncbi.nlm.nih.gov/pmc/articles/PMC3222258/.

Houghton, M. (2019, December). NIH. "Hepatitis C Virus: 30 Years After Discovery." https://www.ncbi.nlm.nih.gov/pmc/articles/PMC6886456/.

Hurum, J. (n.d.). National Geographic. "Nov. 24,1974 CE; Lucy Discovered in Africa." https://education.nationalgeographic.org/resource/lucy-discovered-africa.

KFF. (2022, December 20). "Health Coverage of Immigrants." https://www.kff.org/racial-equity-and-health-policy/fact-sheet/health-coverage-and-care-of-immigrants/.

Koch, M.R. (2021, November). *NIH National Library of Medicine.* "The Frequency of Unnecessary Testing in Hospitalized Patients." https://www.ncbi.nlm.nih.gov/pmc/articles/PMC8628817/.

Lab Pulse. (2021, September 27). "Beckman Coulter Launches DxU Iris." https://www.labpulse.com/diagnostic-technologies/article/15289810/beckman-coulter-launches-dxu-iris-urinalysis-system-at-aacc#:~:text=DxU%20Iris%20is%20designed%20to,%25%2C%20according%20to%20the%20company.

Ledford, H. (2000, October 19). *Nature.* "The Unsung Hero of the Winning Hep C Discovery." https://www.nature.com/articles/d41586-020-02932-y.

Levinson, H.A. (2022, November 3). *Health Costs.* "Hospital Charity Care: How It Works and Why It Matters." https://www.kff.org/health-costs/issue-brief/hospital-charity-care-how-it-works-and-why-it-matters/.

Lim, G. (2014, December 14). *Nature Reviews; Cardiology.* "Warfarin: From Rat Poison to Clinical Use." https://www.nature.com/articles/nrcardio.2017.172#:~:text=The%20discovery%20of%20warfarin%20originated,bleeding%20with%20no%20obvious%20cause.

Mayo Clinic. (1998–2022). *Mayo Clinic.* "Hemochromotosis." https://www.mayoclinic.org/diseases-conditions/hemochromatosis/symptoms-causes/syc-20351443#:~:text=Hereditary%20hemochromatosis%20is%20caused%20by,far%20the%20most%20common%20type.

Mayo Clinic. (2021, July 22). *Mayo Clinic.* "Hemolytic Uremic Syndrome." https://www.mayoclinic.org/diseases-conditions/hemolytic-uremic-syndrome/symptoms-causes/syc-20352399.

Merck. (2022, September). *Merck Manual for Professionals.* "Normal Laboratory Values." https://www.merckmanuals.com/professional/resources/normal-laboratory-values/blood-tests-normal-values.

MSF. (2023). *Our Work.* MSF USA: Doctors Without Borders/Médecins Sans

Frontières (MSF) cares for people affected by conflict, disease outbreaks, natural and human-made disasters, and exclusion from healthcare in more than 70 countries. Independent, impartial medical humanitarian assistance.

NIH. (2022, November 17). *NIH National Cancer Institute.* "Division of Cancer Control and Population Science: Statistics." https://cancercontrol.cancer.gov/ocs/statistics.

Petri, W.J. (2022, September). *Merck Manual.* "Ehrlichiosis and Anaplasmosis." https://www.merckmanuals.com/home/infections/rickettsial-and-related-infections/ehrlichiosis-and-anaplasmosis.

Quicken. (2015, December 21). "Childcare Costs Vs. Income." https://www.quicken.com/blog/child-care-costs-vs-income/#:~:text=Budget%20Guidelines%20for%20Daycare,percent%20of%20a%20household's%20budget.

Rakshit, M.A. (2023). *Peterson-KFF Health Tracker.* "How Does US Expectancy Compare to Other Countries." https://www.healthsystemtracker.org/chart-collection/u-s-life-expectancy-compare-countries/#Life%20expectancy%20at%20birth%20in%20years,%201980-2021.

Reed, B. (2022, January 9). *The Guardian.* "Global Spread of Autoimmune Diseases Blamed on Western Diet." https://www.theguardian.com/science/2022/jan/08/global-spread-of-autoimmune-disease-blamed-on-western-diet.

Savelieff, M. (2018, June 25). *Terchnology Network.* "Clinical Microbiology Id by MALDi Tof ." https://www.technologynetworks.com/immunology/articles/clinical-microbial-identification-by-maldi-tof-mass-spectrometry-303222.

Sompayrac, L. (2012). *How the Immune System Works.* Hoboken, NJ: Wiley-Blackwell.

Stone, J. (2022, April 28). *Forbes.* "We're Facing a Critical Shortage of Medical Laboratory Professionals." https://www.forbes.com/sites/judystone/2022/04/28/were-facing-a-critical-shortage-of-medical-laboratory-professionals/?sh=3161f6b260c2.

Thompson, D. (2023, January 16). *US News.* "Hundreds of Hospitals Could Close Across Rural America." https://www.usnews.com/news/health-news/articles/2023-01-16/hundreds-of-hospitals-could-close-across-rural-america#:~:text=More%20than%20200%20rural%20hospitals,and%20Payment%20Reform%20report%20states.

United Nations Population Fund. (2022, February). "Female Genital Mutilation FAQ." https://www.unfpa.org/resources/female-genital-mutilation-fgm-frequently-asked-questions.

Viatcheslav, W. (2014, July 30). *Brain Bloggerr.* Vitamin B12 Deficiency in Neurological Conditions." https://brainblogger.com/2014/07/30/vitamin-b12-deficiency-and-its-neurological-consequences/.

Vincenzo, F.M. (2022, March 9). *K Health.* "How Much Does Blood Work Cost in 2022." https://khealth.com/learn/healthcare/how-much-does-bloodwork-cost/.

WHO. (2022). "Malaria." https://www.who.int/health-topics/malaria#tab=tab_1.

Willock, C. (1974). *Africa's Rift Valley.* Amsterdam: Time-Life International.

Wu, A.H. (2006, March 27). *A Selected History and Future of Immunoassay Development and Applications in Clinical Chemistry.* Nat. Laboratory of Medicine, PubMed. gov: https://pubmed.ncbi.nlm.nih.gov/16701599/.

Index

Index

Index